You Can LIVE!

ALL NEW SECOND EDITION

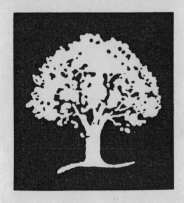

By

Lindsey Williams

YOU CAN LIVE PUBLICATIONS
KASILOF, ALASKA

About the Author

Lindsey Williams has been an ordained minister for over thirty-five years. He was first introduced to health-conscious living through the scriptures and has personally practiced and advocated healthy living for years.

In 1980, Mr. Williams authored his first book, which was to become a bestseller. Since his first book, he has authored numerous others.

Lindsey Williams is an accomplished lecturer and has traveled extensively in America and abroad.

The writing goal of Mr. Williams always has been to seek out the truth. "Ye shall know the truth and the truth shall make you free," is one of his favorite quotations from the scriptures.

Contents

Introduction

Gradually, we are seeing progress in the treatment and prevention of illness and disease in America. Many *bona fide,* licensed physicians—AMA-approved MDs—are beginning to recognize the benefits provided by certain alternative health care, nutritional supplements, and other options available to replace or augment traditional treatments.

Empirical, scientific investigations, with double-blind studies, have been conducted and revealed that there is, in fact, much value in substances and treatments heretofore considered quackery. I, for one, am excited to see this attitude of open-mindedness beginning to surface on the medical scene in America, even though we are considerably behind Europe and the Orient in the acceptance of new—and in many cases, old—methods of successful medical treatment.

God gives us a clear plan in His Word about health and nutrition, but the majority of people choose to ignore it. The Bible tells us what foods are good for us...as well as which are not. It tells us that the herbs of the field and the "leaves of the tree were for the healing of the nations," God's own prescription medicine. Now, I would have to think it would be mighty hard to improve on God's personal prescription.

I have been lecturing on ways to improve our health for a number of years now, and one of the things I've discovered is that even if we try to eat the right foods, the soil is so depleted that the nutrients in our food are mostly nonexistent. Therefore, we must learn what supplements our bodies require in the way of vitamins and minerals, how to prepare our food in utensils that are safe, how to eliminate toxic substances from our bodies, how to clean out our systems (all the way down to the cellular level), how to get sufficient oxygen to those cells for proper metabolism and waste removal, and much more.

I am convinced this book will help you accomplish that goal, and I wholeheartedly recommend the products and health care described herein.

The chapters in this book were written by the authors listed, and they assume full responsibility for the content and its accuracy. To the best of my knowledge, the material is true and without error.

Chapter 1

Medicine for The Next Century

By Arthur R. Davis, Jr., M.D.

What an intriguing thought! Pulling back the curtain of the future and looking at what will be. Exciting to consider, isn't it? There are many benefits to exploring this subject. By becoming aware of what the future holds, you can utilize the experiences and technology to your advantage.

In the following pages, you will find several ideas. These are meant to whet your appetite. They also will acquaint you with some of the technology that exists today, as well as prepare you for what is on the horizon. Enjoy as we explore together!

Philosophy

To better understand the medicine of the future, it would be advantageous to understand where we are today. Currently, the practice of medicine is in a state of major change. In the past, it was simply a doctor/patient encounter. For example, if you came down with a sore throat, you would go to your physician, describe the problem, and request a treatment to cure the problem. This usually would be given as some type of medication. You would pay for the service and leave. Today, because of multiple factors, such as managed health care (HMO), the cost of medication, people's increased interest in their own health and prevention of disease, and government involvement in medicine, the scenario is very different. Now, instead of just requesting medication from your doctor, several other questions often are asked. "What's wrong with me?" "How did I get this?" "How long will it take to get over this?" And most important, "What can I do to prevent this from happening again?"

As you can see, the questions are changing. This represents a major shift in the attitude of the patient. Rather than wanting someone else to just fix the problem, people are far more interested in being involved with their own care—understanding what the problem is, helping to minimize the problem, and even preventing it from recurring. The focus then shifts from "What can you do for me?" to "How can I help myself?"

In the future, there will be a further shift in responsibility from doctor to patient. The patient's emphasis then will become, "How do I treat myself when this problem occurs, so I don't have to visit the doctor?" or even better, "What can I do to prevent this from occurring again?" As well as an emphasis on prevention, people also will be interested much more in natural ways of treating themselves and preventing illness, because the cost is much less, the risk of side effects is much less, and they can care for themselves in the comfort and convenience of their own home.

The role of physicians (of whatever discipline) will shift from being treating therapists to becoming educators; from treating a disease to educating patients about the disease and natural ways to treat, or better yet, prevent it.

What this represents to you, the consumer, is *great opportunity!* It will be a chance for you to have much greater control of your medical care in all areas, from prevention through treatment. There will be increasingly better tools to enable you to learn about—and then care for—your and your family's health.

To further understand what the future has in store for us, let's take a look at how medical practitioners view health and disease today. Then we will explore what changes will be occurring. Let's first examine how we view disease in today's environment, according to Webster's definition, disease is "An impairment of the normal state of the living animal. . .or any of its components that interrupts or modifies the performance of vital functions. . . ." Simply stated, one could say, "Disease is what occurs when things in the body aren't working right." This, of course, is the simple part. What is challenging, first of all, is to understand *why* things aren't working right, and then to determine what part of today's response is good/helpful and what part is bad/harmful. To illustrate, let's suppose that right after a rich, holiday feast you become ill with symptoms of fever, runny nose, chest congestion, and generalized aching. Traditionally, this would be diagnosed as either the flu (viral infection) or maybe bronchitis and treated with a decongestant or cough syrup, or perhaps an antibiotic if it was felt that a bacterial infection was present. The causative agent would be either a virus or a bacteria. You also might be given medication for pain and/or fever. No one would dispute the fact that you were sick; however, it could be hotly disputed what specifically caused the illness and which symptoms are harmful or which are just your body's response to the offending problem. Rather than carry these questions further, let me share with you my perspective on the future of medical care. Medical practitioners will become much more knowledgeable about what leads to the disease state, therefore, effective prevention can be instituted. This will become particularly important in the areas of degenerative disease such as cancer, heart disease, arthritis, etc. We also will become much more knowledgeable about the body's process of fighting disease AND how to assist it in doing so.

As to health—the second part of the equation—Webster defines it: "The condition of an organism or one of its parts in which it performs the vital functions normally or properly." Most people would agree with this definition—or at least one would think so. However, aren't there different levels of normal function—even for you? Consider this: If you contrast how your body functions when you are eating with how it functions when you are climbing five flights of stairs, "normal" function is quite different. It depends upon the activity in which you are participating. Suppose you decide to train for a marathon and are successful in doing so. Normal function will be markedly different if you compare it when you first started training with when you completed training. Wouldn't you agree? You can see that Webster's definition leaves a lot to be desired, especially when you realize that most people consider themselves to be healthy when they are not sick. I have news for you—GREAT NEWS!—enter a new technology called functional complementary medicine.

With this, your health is not defined just as lack of disease, or even normal function (whatever that may be). This new way of looking at things assesses how your body is functioning in many different areas and assesses what your needs are (nutritional, etc.). Then it monitors you as you work toward obtaining "optimal" function. Sounds exciting, doesn't it! The important truth that I wish to emphasize is that functional complementary medicine is not a futuristic technology. It is here now. It is being used by numerous physicians and practitioners even as you read this chapter. Let me share with you the views of Dr. Roy E. Vartabedian, Dr.P.H., M.P.H., F.A.P.C.A., a preventive care specialist.

MEDICINE FOR THE NEXT CENTURY

By Dr. Roy E. Vartabedian

Modern medicine today is predominantly disease-oriented. In the future, medicine finally will shift toward preventive medicine.

Medicine in the next century undoubtedly will be more high-tech, but it will retain its "high touch," as people always will need the "art" part of medicine, as well as the science. Medicine is a "human" science, therefore, it cannot become a mere technology.

Medicine will become more global, just as every other aspect of our lives is becoming. Financially, with the linking of world markets, we see the trend. With the news media, such as CNN, we see the world now. As technology and the information super-highway develop, shared medical knowledge from anywhere in the world will be at our fingertips.

Medicine is coming home to self-help care. More and more home tests will be developed so we can monitor our health, before it is too late.

Managed care will continue to force cost-containment. As a result, it finally will be realized that it is cheaper and more cost-effective to maintain good health than it is to regain it, once it is lost. Presently, we spend 97% of our health-care dollars to treat disease, and in many cases to prolong death, not life. We cannot do this much longer because of the tremendous cost of extending life indefinitely through traditional medicine. Dr. C. Everett Koop stated last year [1994] that prevention can postpone up to 70% of all premature deaths, while traditional medicine postpones only 10-15%.

Evolution or Revolution?

In the early 1960's and previous to this, preventive medicine was treatment-oriented and revolved around treatment modalities, and increasing knowledge or skills related to the treatment. From this, we evolved to include more information on the disease itself, as patients became more interested in the disease process and how to prevent it from occurring.

The next evolutionary leg was moving on to health promotion, because now patients want to get further into the root of the problem and actually promote health, rather than know about the disease or treatment process.

Treatment Education ► Disease Education ► Health Promotion

Within the area of health promotion, there has been another evolution. In general, this evolution has gone from health promotion of the body, or the physical realm, to more recently, the area of the mind and the psychological realm. Again, looking back to the early 60's, it began with the U.S. Surgeon General's Report on Smoking and Health in 1964. This effort was geared toward prevention of a specific disease, namely lung cancer, but the health promotion emphasis was on smoking cessation.

Later, in the same decade around 1968, the exercise boom began to take shape. Leaders in the area, such as Dr. Kenneth H. Cooper and Dr. George Sheehan, as well as others, promoted the idea that exercise not only could prevent disease, but also promote health and well-being.

Just as the exercise boom began gaining momentum in the early 70's, the nutrition emphasis took a stronghold on Americans. People began to realize that although exercise could compensate for some of the negative effects of diet and other bad health habits, optimal nutrition was necessary to achieve a full measure of good health. All three emphases related to health promotion in the area of the physical body.

In the early 80's, we began to see a strong interest in the area of stress management and the major influences of the mind on the body. I believe many of the next major advances in health promotion will be the psychological influences of the mind on the body, as we look at stress and its negative effects, as well as the state of mental health and psychological well-being on various parameters, such as immunological functions. Already, research in this area is mounting to show us an incredible mind-body connection, and how our mental state and outlook feed back to our body functions and the disease—or prevention of disease—processes.

Disease ► Exercise ► Nutrition ► Stress Management ► Psychological Influences
◄   **BODY**   ►   ◄   **MIND**   ►

This all may sound complicated, but as complex as all the research may sound, it all boils down to how we live—the basic health habits of our existence—that influences our health more than anything else. Dr. Lester Breslow, in a classic study of health habits such as diet, exercise, proper weight, moderation, etc. of 9,000 people followed for 10 years, concluded that, "The daily habits of people have a great deal more to do with what makes them sick and when they die than all the influences of medicine." The study showed that if most of the health habits he studied were followed, men could live 11 years longer and women 7 years longer, and they could look and feel 10 to 20 years younger throughout their lives.

What You Can Do

The following is a summary of key health habits that I believe will help you prevent disease and promote optimal health:

1. Exercise between 30 and 60 minutes per day, 5 to 6 days per week at a moderate pace. This includes walking, bicycling, swimming, aerobic dance, etc. Exercise outdoors when possible to receive fresh air and sunlight each day. Use an air purifier indoors if air quality is in question.

2. Eat the most nutrient-dense per calorie foods from each of the following food groups each day: vegetables, fruits, whole grains, legumes, low or non-fat milk/dairy, lean fish/poultry/meat. Talk with your doctor about new medical advances regarding nutritional supplements, and use those specifically prescribed for your condition.

3. Be aware of stresspoints in your life and your body. Back off when these points are passed and practice stress management/relaxation techniques.

4. Control blood cholesterol, triglycerides, glucose, uric acid,

and blood pressure to your doctor's recommendation.

   5. Be cigarette smoke-free.

   6. Be alcohol-free.

   7. Drink 6 to 8 glasses of filtered (purified) water daily. Add one glass for every 30 minutes of exercise, or each hour in hot weather outdoors.

   8. Get 7 to 8 hours of sleep per night.

   9. Develop the mental aspect of your life, including: increase your knowledge base continually, spiritual development and contact with higher power, relationship development and maintenance, fulfilling your purpose in life through your work and in helping others.

More of the Future

   Preventive medicine and health promotion have evolved and will continue to evolve. Americans' view of health has changed dramatically over recent years. Health is not defined by minimal standards anymore, such as the "absence of disease." It is becoming clear that optimal health goes beyond this to a state of "total well-being," creating a large buffer zone between sickness and health, while dramatically increasing "quality of life."

   As much as the advances of medicine will propel us to a greater quality of life and an increase in longevity, how we live our lives (how we eat, drink, sleep, work, and think) will affect us more than any other factor. Our daily choices will impact our lives (including how much we decide to utilize all of the new medical advances) more than all the influences of medicine. Yes, we still will be in control of our own destiny, for the most part. When we die, we die not from the disease itself, but from the choices of our entire life.

   The diseases from which we will be most likely to die are—and will continue to be—"lifestyle" diseases, primarily heart disease, cancer, stroke, diabetes, hypertension, obesity, hyperlipidemia, and arthritis. These diseases have no "cure," other than a change in the cause. . .which is how we live. There never will be a "pill" that we can take to change the fact that we are couch-potatoes, or that we eat whatever we want. All of the positive physiological changes which come about from exercise, proper nutrition, and a balanced mental state never will be able to be simulated; the real thing always will be the best (and cheapest) way to go.

Time will become more precious; time with family, time for leisure activities, time for hobbies and pursuit of personal goals, and time away from the pressures of our fast-paced society will be at a premium. Many have realized that without good health, this time is useless, so personal motivation for health promotion will increase. We already have seen the tip of the iceberg with the proliferation of health clubs, exercise equipment, nutritional supplements, stress-reducers, and home-health screening tools.

Life expectancy will continue to increase into the 21st Century. Man's lifespan theoretically can be increased to a potential 120 years. But who wants to live longer if the **quality** of life is not there with the **quantity** of life?

For this, I will leave you with the statement from Ern Baxter, from his book, *I Almost Died,* "If your lifestyle does not control your body, eventually your body will control your lifestyle." I feel that Ern's words always will be true—even into the 21st Century and beyond.

Roy E. Vartabedian, Dr.P.H., M.P.H., F.A.P.C.A., is a preventive care specialist in private practice with Arthur R. Davis, M.D., near Palm Springs, California. He is author of the international best-seller, *Nutripoints: The Breakthrough Program for Optimal Nutrition,* which utilizes a unique point system to evaluate foods based on computer analyses of 26 nutritional factors.

What the future will hold is more and better tests that will enable your physicians to understand more fully the source of your body's lack of health at a cellular level and assist them in helping you to correct the problem! In summary, regarding health and disease: the emphasis in the future will shift from a focus of treatment of symptoms and disease entities to a much better understanding of how your body works, what it needs to work better, and how best to supply that.

How to Choose a Physician

Choosing a physician is a particularly important issue for the next century. I believe what we will see is a much stronger position for the natural healing arts as time goes on. This is already the case in Europe, where homeopathy, aromatherapy, manipulative therapies, diet therapies, etc., have been in use for some time and have professional standing in the medical community. Therefore, it will be important for you to be very clear about what you require in a physician. Here are some suggestions that will help you.

• Do you want your physician to allow you to participate in the decision-making process? If so, tell him/her in the beginning of your relationship what you expect.

• Do you want a physician with whom you can share yourself? If so, make certain he/she listens to you.

• Do you want a physician who will consider alternative/non-traditional therapies? Even if he isn't knowledgeable, ask him if he will be willing to monitor you as you treat yourself (more about this in the next section, "How to Educate Your Physician").

• Do you want a physician who will inform you about what is going on and what you can do to make a difference? Share with him how important this is to you.

• Do you want a physician with a user-friendly office? When you first talk with him, ask him with whom you should talk if you have a problem.

These are just a few questions to ask, but they will help you get clear in your mind which physician is the one you want as part of the team that will help you make your life run more smoothly. Remember, we live in a free enterprise society, and the choice is yours. So exercise that responsibility carefully.

How to Educate Your Physician

Suppose you have a physician you really like. He listens, he's kind, gentle, and understanding...but either he doesn't know or *doesn't want to know* about something related to your health care that is very important to you. Is there a way to keep him as your physician and, yet, make him an integral part of your health team? I believe there is, and I'd like to tell you how.

To explain how this works, I first must share some important information with you. Physicians, by nature, are inquisitive people. They like to know how and why things work as they do. They also get very excited when they know that they are helping people and making a difference in their lives. They often get very

interested when they see a patient getting better, even if they just
are monitoring the patient while he or she does their own therapy.
You see, it really isn't all that hard to involve them in your
progress...and then educate them. Here is how it is done.

1. Tell them you're starting something new for your problem,
and you need their help. This may lead to a few raised eyebrows.

2. Quickly add that what you need from them is for them to
monitor you and your progress, and ask if they will do that.

3. While you are treating yourself, write down what you are
doing and keep progress notes. (Charts and graphs are very
helpful.)

4. Show these charts, graphs, and notes to your physician and
ask what he thinks. (Be prepared to share in detail what you
are doing.)

5. As your physician gets interested, have scientific literature
available (the best you can get), but *give only one piece at a time*.

6. When your physician is *really* interested, have a professional
available with whom he can talk regarding the therapy program
you are following.

7. Always maintain an attitude of gratitude and humility and
enthusiasm.

8. Expect it to work and usually it will—patience is critical!

The Role of Traditional Medicine in Our Society

We will define traditional or "mainstream" medicine as that
form of medicine that is sanctioned by the American Medical
Association (AMA) and is practiced in virtually all hospitals
and the majority of medical doctors' offices today. It is primarily
disease-oriented, heavily focused on symptom control or relief,
and is supported by the majority of consumers in America today.

"What's wrong with it?" you ask. Several things—it's far too
expensive; the focus is very heavy on treatment, rather than
prevention; and it really doesn't get at the cause of most of
today's diseases. Are there other problems? Yes, many other
problems, but I have listed just the major ones.

What's good about it? Several things—it is excellent medicine
in crisis situations; it is very helpful in dealing with disease states
that are out of control, such as overwhelming infections, acute
psychiatric problems, terminal illnesses, advanced endocrine
disorders, trauma, etc.

What is the role of traditional medicine in the future? It will continue to be extremely important in crisis medicine (trauma, breakdowns, etc.). It has some very hopeful genetic advances on the horizon for treating such things as cystic fibrosis and diabetes mellitus, to name a few. Surgical techniques are advancing rapidly and will lead to less and less invasive procedures. All this suggests that with the advent of managed health care, the future of traditional medicine can be helpful, more cost-effective, and increasingly user-friendly for you.

The Role of Nontraditional Medicine in Society Today

In the category of nontraditional medicine, we place everything that is not considered traditional/allopathic medicine. This covers a very broad range that not even an entire book could cover, let alone part of a chapter. What is really important, however, is the role that these branches of the healing arts play now and will play in the future.

We already have discussed functional/complementary medicine, in brief. It is critical to the success of all forms of alternative therapies. The bottom line is not only how a person *feels,* but what his *function* is. Functional/complementary medicine will help support *objectively* what is occurring *subjectively* in the body.

A very strong "positive" for alternative healing is its emphasis on identifying the cause of the problem and dealing with it. Disease, then, is looked at not as a specific set of symptoms, but rather as a disordered set of systems (digestive, cardiac, endocrine, respiratory, etc.), why they aren't working properly, and what can be done to correct them.

In the future, this type of medical practice will continue to improve in determining causes, particularly of the degenerative diseases, and give the patient better ways of correcting the underlying problems *and* enhancing optimal function.

Technology

How would you like an information and resource center that you could call, fax, or write to obtain information regarding the numerous alternatives available that traditional and nontraditional medicine offer you today? Wouldn't it be great to have one central data center where all this information is available? Well,

it will be now. With the birth of this chapter came the birth of
that concept. It is my plan to form an organization to act as
a clearing house resource center for this kind of information all
over the United States of America and, probably later, all over
the world. This would provide you with ready access to all that
is available to enhance your health and well-being for just a
nominal fee.

This is a small part of where technology will go in the future.
Computers will assist us in all kinds of ways. For instance, I
believe it won't be long before a patient can walk into his doctor's
office and access his own records, then educate himself by
computer as to what he can do to improve his health. Another
advancement will be the rise of much better health networks,
so that when you go from place to place, your kind of health
care and provider will be available to you readily, along with your
records.

Technology represents opportunity, if used correctly. Since the
health field is based so heavily on information, I believe advancing technology will represent *major* opportunity!

Tools for Enhancing Your Own Health

1. Nutripoints—a system for eating to maximize your nutrition.
2. Medicine for the next century resource center—information
about places and people and things and unique healing
techniques.
3. Nutritional counseling—a conversation with a nutritionist,
so you can understand better what your body needs and how
you can maximize your nutrients.
4. Physical conditioning counseling—consulting a conditioning expert who can understand the uniqueness of your body and
structure a program specifically tailored to your needs.
5. Relaxation techniques—learning how to allow your body
truly to rest, relax, and rebuild.
6. Spiritual enhancement—finding ways to center your life
around its most important part, and thereby enhance the meaning and significance of your journey through life.
7. Habits assessment—What do you do habitually that either
makes you healthy or unhealthy?—and what do you want to do
about it?
8. Water intake evaluation—Is the water you drink pure and

wholesome, or do you need purified or distilled water to enhance your health?

9. Mental evaluation—What is your mental function? Can you do things to make a difference today, such as changing your focus?

10. Stretching exercises—These will enhance your ability to get about, decrease your pain, and improve your sense of well-being.

11. Scripture for the Christian—There are many tremendous promises to enhance your health and aid in the healing process.

Summary

As you readily can see, medicine for the next century offers a wide variety of great opportunities! You will have a much better understanding of your body and the laws that govern it. You will understand what causes disease, how you best can treat it, how to prevent it, and—most important—how to maximize your health.

You will be able to pick the physician or health care specialist you like and educate the one you already have. You will have access to a resource bank of information to help you find the treatment and health care program you like best.

Computers will enable you to access information about yourself, so you can assist more easily in your own healing.

The Nutripoint system can enhance your eating enjoyment, while at the same time allowing you to become nutritionally fit.

Remember, your first day of the next century is today. Make it your best day ever and keep building on it. May you have the very best health, happiness, and spiritual well-being!

Arthur R. Davis, Jr., M.D.

Dr. Davis is a busy general practitioner who loves people and enjoys teaching them how to live healthier lives. He has quite a varied background, ranging from a general practice in Lake Arrowhead, California, to working with Dr. Virginia Livingston (a physician who developed an immune vaccine to treat cancer), to running a nutritional program at American International Hospital in Zion, Illinois, to a very busy general practice in the desert area of Blythe, California. Currently, he is located in the Palm Springs, California, area and is involved heavily in managed health care. His greatest interest, however, is assisting people to become more healthy, using natural, as well as traditional medicine. He is co-authoring a book with Dr. Vartabedian entitled *How to Enjoy Livin' Life,* and also is organizing a resource center for people interested in information and materials about all forms of healing.

— RESPONSE PAGE —

☐ I am very interested in your organization that will provide me with information about various types of healing alternatives throughout the United States. Please send me information regarding this as soon as possible.

☐ I am very interested in information about Dr. R. Vartabedian's Nutripoints program. Please send me information regarding this as soon as possible.

Please make your selection(s) and send to:

Arthur R. Davis, Jr., M.D.
81-709 Dr. Carreon Blvd., Ste. C-5,6
Indio, CA 92201

Phone: (619) 347-7730
Fax: (619) 342-3001

Chapter 2

The Immune System— Under Attack and Defending

By Terry S. Friedmann, M.D.,(H)

Our world presents a hostile environment that increasingly stresses and weakens our immune system, our primary line of defense against disease. We must be cognizant of the dangers confronting us. In the following pages it will be revealed to you how you may nourish and strengthen your immune system, as well as how to reverse acute and chronic debilitating diseases. A five-step program, developed by me, will assist you in achieving good health.

Infectious Diseases

Today, a large number of environmental stresses are attacking our body's immune system. Because of these stresses and the sudden emergence of new and highly virulent infectious diseases, our health is being challenged severely.

New viruses are attacking us constantly. Every year millions of people contract the flu, and many die as a consequence of its complications. One reason the flu is difficult to prevent and cure is that the virus mutates radically every year, forming new strains. The Marburg virus outbreak caused infected victims to suffer a painful death by internal bleeding, attacking the nervous system and stomach.

Recently, the news media reported an infection similar to the Marburg virus—it was the deadly Ebola viral infection that broke out in Zaire, Africa. And why are these viruses so dreaded? Simple! When one is infected, one has a 90% chance of becoming a fatality statistic. Authorities from the World Health Organization rushed to Zaire in an effort to contain the deadly virus and stop it from spreading to other countries.

With airline travel so readily available to the mass population —whether they live in the Amazon or Africa—someone who contracted a virus in a foreign nation literally could be in New York City the same day they became infected with the deadly germ. In addition, with the continuous recycling of the oxygen on airliners, every passenger and crew member could contract the disease, or become a carrier. With many passengers transferring to other planes to reach their final destination, the potential for starting a widespread epidemic not only exists, but seems inevitable.

However, it is not only these new viruses about which we should be concerned. Old diseases, in recent years considered extinct illnesses from our past, are again rearing their ugly heads and threatening to cause new epidemics. These include diphtheria, cholera, anthrax, tuberculosis, and "the plague." Both in medieval Europe and as late as the early 1900's, we were led to believe that these germs were a problem only because of inadequate sanitation and poor personal hygiene. Even though both of these contribute to the spread of disease, it has been discovered that they are not the exclusive cause of the problem. Of course, antibiotics had not yet been discovered to aid in the control of such diseases previous to this century.

Gratefully, with the advance of antibiotics, many of these diseases were cured, and some all but obliterated. However, because of the widespread and inexcusable overuse of antibiotics, many infectious organisms have developed resistant strains. Many of these new strains cannot be killed with our existing antibiotics. Tuberculosis is a good example of the appearance of a new, highly resistant strain of this organism and has baffled doctors and other scientists during the last 15 years.

Even our water supplies—upon which we are so dependent because they are critical to our health and well-being—are becoming contaminated in some of America's largest cities. A serious outbreak of gastroenteritis occurred after the intestinal parasite *Cryptosporidium parvum* was found in the municipal drinking water of one city in 1993. Hundreds of people sought treatment at hospital emergency rooms, and many died because of compromised immune systems. Now, we are finding these same parasites in the drinking water of other large American cities, including New York and Phoenix.

Also, we just now are learning that the common gastric and duodenal ulcer is not caused merely by improper lifestyle, as previously thought. Actually, it was found that as high as 92% of duodenal ulcers are caused primarily by an infectious bacteria called *Heliobacter pylori*. This is a corkscrew-shaped bacteria that invades the gastrointestinal mucosa and secretes urease that, in turn, produces ammonia. This protects the bacteria against the effects of hydrochloric acid, which is secreted by the stomach to digest food. By neutralizing this acid, the bacteria is able to survive. Of course, this disrupts our digestion process.

One illness that exemplifies the complete failure of the immune system is AIDS. The HIV virus invades the immune system and suppresses and cripples its function, limiting the body's ability to fight off infections. As we know, this usually ends in death. Without a cure, this disease is infecting more and more of the population, and the fact that it is spreading rapidly into all areas of every population is well publicized.

Environmental Toxins

Inorganic toxins are another major cause of a depressed immune system. You frequently hear of toxins in our environment (air, soil, and food pollution) and the harm that they can do. Much is written about them and their effects, but most of us believe they can't really affect us all that seriously.

However, we only have to look at what has happened to our major cities over the last several years. A dirty haze settles over them, and the Department of Environmental Quality has determined that air quality has reached unhealthful proportions in many cities. The reason cited is a major warm air/cold air inversion, trapping the pollution produced by wood-burning stoves and fireplaces, aerosol sprays, and thousands of cars. The increase in traffic is caused, of course, by the tremendous population growth in most of our major cities.

This problem is expected to continue, but the question is, "What are the physical consequences of air pollution?" Some people experience burning, itching, and infected eyes, sore throat, and bronchial cough, which could lead to serious respiratory infections, as well as an increase in asthma, bronchitis, and pneumonia conditions.

Then there is the petro-chemical exposure in our environment; the amount of pesticides, herbicides, and other chemicals applied to our crops and landscaping is very high. The Environmental Protection Agency estimates that two pounds per acre of these products are added to our food crops yearly, five pounds to our neatly groomed lawns, and 15 to 40 pounds per acre of chemicals are applied to our golf courses annually.

According to the National Institute of Health, groundskeepers and managers of country clubs suffer from three times the incidence of lymphoma than the general population. Persons living on golf courses also have an increased risk of cancer and other diseases.

We also may see serious neurological effects from these petro-chemical toxins. These may include fever, nausea, weakness, tremors, flushing of the skin, dullness of concentration and thought, pounding heart, and numbness in the hands and feet.

Many of us also have been exposed to large amounts of heavy metals, such as mercury, lead, aluminum, and cadmium, all of which interfere with the health of our immune systems. In addition, lead may damage the mitochondria that act as power plants for muscles. This causes severe physical weakness and pain.

We must consider the risks involved in drinking water and eating food. Many chemicals are found in these necessary and nourishing products that sustain life.

Our protection and defense against these diseases and toxins is the immune system. How does it work?

The Immune System

The term "immune" comes from the Latin word *immunist* that means "exempt from, resistant to, or protected from disease, infectious organisms, poisons, allergens, and other agents." Our bodies tend to defend themselves against an outside substance or particle that is foreign to them.

In response to stressors (anything causing stress), both physical (chemicals, bacteria, viruses, foods, pollens, or mold) and psychological, our brain releases various substances that assist in the protection of the body.

We have two types of cells that generally react with allergens. These are "T" cells and "B" cells, each a type of antibody. Allergens are any environmental material. They can be inhalants (such as pollens, molds, animal danders, and insect parts), or ingestants (such as foods and drugs), or contactants (such as hair dyes, cosmetics, and metals). Antibodies are proteins produced by the body that protect the body by neutralizing the attacking substance (allergens). When the "T" cell is the mediator (arbitrator or go-between), then we experience a dermal or skin reaction that is an inflammation caused by direct contact. We also can find this type of reaction with an inflammation of the lungs leading to pneumonitis secondary to hypersensitivity to an allergen.

The immune system is stimulated by way of the thymus gland and the bursal equivalent. Products formed by these organs function to counteract the effects of the stressors.

Auto Immunity

Autoimmune diseases cannot be explained by a solitary cause or mechanism. Small amounts of auto-antibodies normally are produced and may have physiological roles in cellular interactions. The major theories regarding the development of autoimmune diseases are (1) release of normal sequestered antigens (a portion of a virus, bacteria, etc.), (2) the presence of abnormal clones, (3) shared antigens between the host and microorganisms, and (4) defects in helper or suppressor cell functions.

Genetic susceptibility is also a likely determinant of autoimmune disease. In nearly all autoimmune diseases, multiple mechanisms of auto immunity are operative, and the exact causes are unknown.

Humoral Antibody-Mediated Auto Immunity

The existence of antireceptor (something that blocks messages to the body's organs) antibodies that compete with or mimic various physiologic antagonists for cellular receptors is a specific autoimmune mechanism in several diseases. In Graves' disease, a thyroid condition, antibodies are present that compete with thyroid cells and stimulate thyroid hormone production. In rare instances of type I diabetes mellitus, anti-insulin receptor antibodies cause insulin resistance in distant tissues.

Immune Complex Disease

With this group of diseases (systemic lupus erythematosus, rheumatoid arthritis, some drug-induced hemolytic anemia, and thrombocytopenia), autologous or similar body tissues are injured as "innocent bystanders."

Support and Repair of Our Immune System

So, what must we do to repair and support our frequently dysfunctional immune system to protect ourselves against an onslaught of infectious diseases and environmental toxins?

I have developed a "5-Step" program, which—if followed—will enable patients to reverse their dysfunctional immune system and illnesses and create health and high-level wellness. I call this program the "5 R's":
1. Remove
2. Replace
3. Repair
4. Rejuvenate
5. Revitalize

Step One—Remove (In this step, "remove" also means to avoid.)

Attempt to avoid toxins by staying indoors on high-pollution days. Also, you must avoid using chemicals and petro-chemically-based sprays in and around your house. Bathe immediately and wash your clothes after playing golf. To neutralize your food, soak and wash your fruit and vegetables thoroughly, using a few drops of household bleach in a quart of water. Eliminate dyes and chemicals from your diet; read food labels. Drink only pure bottled water or, better yet, distilled and filtered water.

Next, we must remove the offending factors. If these factors are heavy metals, such as lead, cadmium, mercury, aluminum, or arsenic, we may chelate them out of the body. This is done by introducing a "chelating agent" into the system that literally grabs the offending material and holds it in solution until the kidneys can flush it out of the system. EDTA (Ethylene Diamine Tetraacetic Acid) is a very fine chelating agent when injected intravenously. EDTA is a protein that binds with all heavy metals and eliminates them safely, excreting them through the kidneys.

An additional benefit is EDTA's ability to find and remove unwanted calcium that often clogs our arteries and impairs our circulation. Opening these arteries also improves the nutrition of body tissues.

DMPS (Dimercapto Propane Sulfonate) is also a powerful chelating agent and has a high affinity for the metal mercury. However, if the factors are primarily pesticides and other chemicals, add to this dry sauna treatments.

If your stomach and bowels are infected with the bacteria *Heliobacter pylori* and other parasites such as protozoa and worms, or yeasts and other fungi, then these must be eliminated. But if the body is already immune-compromised, then safe and natural products must be used instead of damaging antibiotics. I devised such a program using bentonite with colloidal silver that is mild and inoffensive to the body, but is devastating to many parasites and bacteria, including *Heliobacter pylori.*

Sometimes we are allergic to certain foods. These foods may cause injury to the intestinal mucosa. The results could be damaging to the integrity of the filtering system of the mucosa, causing enlargement of these natural openings and admitting large molecular toxins and undigested food. The human digestive system often interprets these large molecules as foreign bodies and reacts in an allergic manner to the food particles. Therefore, once they are identified, these foods must be eliminated from the diet until the immune system is repaired and strengthened.

We also should include in our diet a mixed bran roughage consisting of various grains. These foods mechanically "brush" the intestinal tract, cleansing it of unwanted debris.

I also recommend a highly nutritional three- or five-day fast, under a doctor's care. The fast recommended is the Master Cleanse, using eight to twelve glasses per day of a mixture of:

2 Tbsp. Grade "C" maple syrup
2 Tbsp. freshly squeezed lemon or lime
1/8 tsp. cayenne pepper
8 oz. distilled water

Step Two—Replace

The second step is to replace the products that may be diminished or missing in our gastrointestinal systems. One must reinoculate the intestines. Studies show that in sickness, the bowels usually contain an improper balance of bacterial growth. Over 300 species of beneficial bacteria grow symbiotically (working together in harmony) in our intestinal tract.

Another very important process in the "replacing" step is to assure that you have adequate enzymes for food digestion and assimilation of the nutrients. The major enzymes are pancreatin, lipase, trypsin, and hydrochloric acid. This is only a partial list of enzymes. It should be understood that many of the "B" vitamins are converted by these enzymes, along with the normal intestinal bacteria, into a usable form of Vitamin B, which is so necessary for your body's proper metabolism, growth, and energy.

It is very important to assure that your body has adequate glutathione, a tripeptide that functions in the liver. Glutathione detoxifies and neutralizes chemical products that cause damage to the body. These are called xerobiotics, e.g. any foreign products that are chemically unfriendly to the body. Assuring adequate glutathione protects the body against these products and reverses the aging process.

Step Three—Repair

Now that the digestive and detoxification systems are in place, repair must be performed. The end products of metabolism (waste and debris) must be removed. This must be initiated using antioxidants and free-radical scavengers. These are Vitamins A, C, and E, selenium (a trace mineral), and pycnogenol. The latter is known as a powerful product derived from either grape seed extract or the bark of a pine tree that grows in northern France. These products not only should be taken as a function of this "repair" process, but also as elements of a maintenance program to protect the body.

Participating in this rebuilding process are the nutrients that are the building blocks of the body. These include minerals, both macro and micronutrients—basically encompassing all of the minerals. This, of course, excludes the heavy metals such as lead, cadmium, aluminum, and mercury that may interfere with, rather than support, metabolism of the structures.

Another class of necessary building blocks is the amino acids. These basic proteins are the essential foundation of body tissue, and many of these biochemical products are found in our systems. Most of the amino acids must be taken orally.

Step Four—Rejuvenate

This implies not only the rejuvenation and regeneration of tissues, but organs as well. One recent finding is the inability of the organs to make adequate hormones when we are under duress, hormones so necessary for body functions to occur properly.

DHEA (dehydroepiandrosterone) is a significant representation of this. It has been called the "mother hormone" because it is the raw material from which estrogen, testosterone, progesterone, and corticosterone are made by our bodies. The DHEA level in the blood reaches its peak at 20 years of age and declines with aging. Studies show that some people have premature low levels of DHEA. These same people often experience loss of energy, declining function, and accelerated aging, as well as an increase in degenerative diseases. Conversely, studies show that having acceptable levels of DHEA can prevent or reverse many diseases.

Dr. Elizabeth Barrett-Connor, M.D., from the University of California School of Medicine in San Diego, found a "48% reduction in cardiovascular disease and a 36% reduction in mortality from any cause" when the DHEA levels were increased to therapeutic levels. According to Dr. Barrett-Connor, the reason for this is that DHEA protects the body by inhibiting the enzyme (glucose-6 phosphate dehydrogenase) which normally accelerates the production of both damaging fatty acids and cholesterol.

Other studies reveal that significant diseases such as cancer, obesity, depression, high blood pressure, diabetes, arthritis, senility, and Alzheimer's disease either can be improved or reversed. There are also studies indicating that DHEA may be significant in improving memory and stimulating the immune system. Other studies taken during weight-loss programs have suggested that DHEA may be of significance in the fat-burning process, possibly by replacing fat with muscle tissue.

The best news is that when taken orally, in prescribed doses, DHEA causes no toxicity. Because DHEA is an unpatentable drug, no major pharmaceutical company is interested in informing us of its value and/or marketing it. It is a prescription drug, and a recent report from the FDA claims that it will become a controlled substance. This means it must be used under the direction of a licensed M.D. and purchased from a registered pharmacist.

I recommend that DHEA blood level be evaluated prior to its administration to determine whether or not there is, indeed, a significant decline of your DHEA level. A lack of DHEA could be the cause of your illness and this is a dramatic and safe therapy available to you.

Second, the regeneration step should include purified tissue extracts such as liver, adrenal, and thyroid. These "extract" doses should be low, or even homeopathic. The latter is defined as a product diluted many times, sometimes resulting in only the molecular energy of the original product existing in distilled water. In either case, the benefit of the tissue extracts are found in their ability to restore and rebuild the organs that are damaged and, hence, not functioning properly. Particularly in the instance of homeopathic remedies, their function may be to act as a "blueprint material"—one that sends a message to the body as to how to rebuild the tissues and organs. In some cases, it furnishes raw material for this function, as well.

When there has been severe damage, I use live-cell therapy. This involves administering the thymus gland cells of an unborn sheep or cow. The effect of this therapy is similar to doing an organ transplant, except that it is non-invasive, safer, and simpler. This rebuilds our own thymus gland, enabling it to function at a beneficial level, instead of its frequently dysfunctional level.

We also can restore greatly the mitochondria of a muscle cell, after it has been damaged by heavy metals and other xerobiotics, particularly petro-chemicals. This damage could lead to severe muscle fatigue and diseases such as fibromyalgia. Adding high doses of the natural product Coenzyme Q_{10} stimulates the activity of the muscles, assisting them to function normally. This also holds true for the heart muscle, stimulating it after it has become damaged, flabby, or poorly functioning. Hence, Co-enzyme Q_{10} may improve the heart's function and may reverse serious debilitating heart disease.

There is a very important therapy to consider in rejuvenation. It involves an intravenous injection of ortho-molecular nutrients, specifically high doses of Vitamin C (in the range of 100,000-150,000 mg.). This is 100% absorbed, unlike oral doses.

It will generate rapid healing and destroy infections from viruses, bacteria, and fungi. The high dose of Vitamin C apparently jump-starts the body and kicks the immune system into high gear. In addition to Vitamin C, essential minerals and Vitamins B's are included and administered simultaneously. Generally, this therapy is given for five consecutive days. The results are phenomenal in many cases.

Step Five—Revitalize

The fifth and last step of this program is to revitalize the body. First of all, we should have a good diet. The diet should consist of many vegetables, whole grains, some whole fruit, and protein from beans and brown rice. If you are not a vegetarian, protein also may come from fish and turkey. Less than 15% of the diet should be from polyunsaturated fats which are not excessively heated. We should reduce or eliminate red meats, fried foods, salt, sugar, and refined and overprocessed foods. It is very important to drink eight or more glasses of *pure* water daily.

Exercise is very important. After approval is obtained from your physician, exercise for at least 20 minutes, four times a week. These exercise periods should be of a strenuous enough nature for you to perspire.

Essential oils are a very significant way to revitalize your body and elevate its function to an improved level. Now that we have everything operating properly, let's take it to high gear. The pure oils can take us there. Oils are one of the earliest forms of medicine. They were used in Egypt 4,000 years ago by the priest-physicians. Today, there is no other medicine with such a high frequency as the oils. We are in the age of energy medicine, and the body normally functions between a range of 50-75 kilohertz (kHz). Disease has frequency of 58 kHz down (cancer is 42 kHz), which is one measurement of energy. To combat disease, we use various products. Drugs have a frequency of 0-10 kHz. Herbs have a frequency of 15-22 kHz. Essential oils have a frequency of 70-320 kHz.

These oils oxygenate and revitalize the body. Oils also have the ability to transport nutrients and micronutrients to the body's tissues and enhance the body's energy. One example is the oil Helichrysum, which when applied externally on the body improves the nervous system, stimulating the brain's synaptic firing of an electrical impulse from one nerve to another. Many of the body's functions generate and utilize electrical energy whose frequencies are measured routinely by an electrocardiogram or electroencephalogram. (These are instruments which measure the heart function and the brain waves, respectively.) The electro-frequencies can be changed by the oils. They balance and raise the energies.

Emotions Translate into the Physical

One important aspect of raising the vitality of a person is to remove negative emotional and mental patterns that they have acquired and replace them with positive, creative patterns. Until this concept is addressed fully, disease cannot be reversed com-pletely, nor can the patient be considered completely healthy. I believe that the entire body is a totally synchronized energy machine; if there is a restriction of energy in a specific region of the body, weakness or breakdown in that area ultimately could occur.

When I began to study patterns in patients, I finally under-stood more about the true cause of disease and health. The negative emotions—such as fear, anger, hatred, jealousy, envy, and prejudices—suppress the spirit and, hence, the very nature of man. The person who is filled with emotions such as these is sick physically, mentally, and *spiritually*. For example, patients who are more "fixed" in their thought and behavior patterns often suffer from arthritis. Rigidity in thoughts creates inflexi-bility in the body. Persons who have pent-up emotions and are under a lot of stress frequently have hypertension, which is unrelieved internal pressure. Interestingly enough, these types of patients seldom develop cancer, which instead seems to be caused by other types of behavior, such as fear of loss or loneliness. Often patients who have difficulty expressing love and other personal feelings have blocked coronary (heart) arteries. At times, these patients may feel unloved, as well.

A relatively new science has emerged in which the way we think and act affects our immune system either positively or negatively. This science is called "Psychoneuroimmunology."

The whole category of immune suppression diseases has to do with a host of issues directed inwardly at the patient's life force. This creates disturbances of the immune system. We know this immune suppression is regulated by a part of the brain called the hypothalamus. It helps to modulate emotions such as joy, happiness, sadness, and anger. We understand that our environment is full of toxins and poisons. However, it is obvious that simply being exposed to these poisonous substances does not necessarily insure that disease will prevail.

Repeatedly, we physicians see several patients in the same family who are subjected to similar problems, yet may have completely different responses and outcomes. One may have a disease; the other may be totally healthy. Generally, the difference lies in their individual attitudes and behaviors. So many of our problems are the result of the inability to release old, suppressed hurts that have occurred in the past. It is these hurts that project from the subconscious as reminders of some actual or perceived injury. This injury lodges in the region of the body that most appropriately relates to the specific emotion. For instance, love has to do with the heart, breast, or bladder—the "giving" glands.

Time and time again, we are told to give up the old hurts and negative emotions. If we do not do this, these emotions clearly could manifest as disease or injury. The body literally starts "taking it out on itself."

On the positive side of health, love is the purest and most important emotion that we can express. Love, taken to its highest form, is the most profound expression of our spiritual selves. At this elevated creation, love is called "unconditional" by some religions, while other religions refer to it as *agape*. Here we love fully, no matter what happens—no "ifs," "ands," or "buts." When love is openly given to others, miracles can happen.

There is a complete lack of condemnation here. We know condemnation of others, as well as self, limits health and healing and creates blocks of negative emotion. Anger, fear, and guilt are some of the most destructive emotions. These cause blocks in the natural energy flow of the body that ultimately could lead to breakdown and disease. The opposite of this is love and forgiveness, and the *expression* of it. Love is the most healing modality known on earth today.

What is the key for diagnosing and releasing these patterns? One effective procedure is hypnotherapy. In competent hands, this process can remove deeply established blocks. Once these blocks have been removed, healing can occur.

There are many physical reasons for a breakdown, such as hereditary weakness, nutritional deficiency, fatigue, and accidents. But they often are linked to a deeper pattern. There is a positive effect from simply recognizing the problem; that is, digging it out of the subconscious and experiencing it at a tolerable, conscious level. Releasing the problem mentally and emotionally likely could cause the physical condition to disappear eventually. As simple as it seems, it works. Similar changes occur with homeopathic remedies, particularly if they are given at higher dilutions. If the right remedy is given, they help to remove the negative emotion.

Obviously, each person must deal with many emotions. Removing these problems one at a time is like peeling away multiple layers of an onion's skin. They unfold, one at a time, until you get down to the sweet, internal part. This healthy inner core is vibrant and complete within itself, free of illness. You have the *freedom* to change negative emotions any time you wish —but always do it with joy. Joy is not only a result of us achieving this balanced center, but a joyful attitude along the way helps in the process of finding that new inner peace, as well.

In summary, this 5-Step Program is very comprehensive. Perhaps in some cases only a portion of the program is necessary to achieve a healthy success. With a strong immune system, we not only are able to prevent, but also to reverse disease. This applies to many diseases, such as cardiovascular diseases, allergies, multiple sclerosis, diabetes, chronic fatigue, arthritis, and cancer.

There is no need to continue to suffer from a chronic debilitating disease! This program works because it is based on firm scientific data and personal experience with these diseases in my practice. The most powerful tool we have to heal ourselves is our **belief system**. Either we believe in the physician and his program, or the physician must believe firmly in his ability to heal someone because of his past successes. The implication is that our degree of belief in something is a good indication as to whether or not the disease process will come to a successful and healthy conclusion.

Terry S. Friedmann, M.D., (H)

Dr. Terry Shepherd Friedmann has been a leader in the field of Holistic medicine for many years. Frustrated with "patching-up" people, in 1978 he co-founded and for 14 years served on the Board of Directors of the American Holistic Medical Association. He studied the effects of cholesterol on humans at the Metabolic Institute of the University of California in San Francisco in 1962 and worked on developing cures for parasites while at the National Institute of Tropical Diseases in Mexico City in 1965. He has lectured extensively and appeared on many radio and TV shows, both in the United States and abroad. He is the author of the book, *Freedom Through Health,* and has written numerous articles for newspapers, magazines, and journals. Dr. Friedmann specialized in treating atherosclerosis, allergies, arthritis, multiple sclerosis, candidiasis, immune dysfunction syndrome, diabetes, parasites, and other degenerative diseases.

He is a Diplomate of the American Board of Chelation Therapy and is currently Medical Director of the Phoenix Health and Medical Center.

Dr. Friedmann can be reached at the Phoenix Health & Medical Center, 10565 N. Tatum Blvd., Suite B-115, Paradise Valley, AZ 85253, Phone (602) 381-0800.

NOTE: This chapter contains excerpts from the book, *Freedom Through Health,* by Terry Shepherd Friedmann, M.D.,(H). This book can be ordered through Harvest Publishing Company, 7031 E. Camelback Rd., Suite 481, Scottsdale, AZ 85251.

— RESPONSE PAGE —

I read about the problems with the immune system in Lindsey Williams' new book, *You Can LIVE!*

Please send me _____ copies of *Freedom Through Health* at USA price of $11.95 + $3.10 shipping and handling per copy.

PLEASE SHIP TO:

Name _____

Street/Box No. _____

City/State/Zip _____

Phone (_____) _____

MAKE CHECKS PAYABLE AND MAIL TO:

HARVEST PUBLISHING COMPANY
7031 E. Camelback Rd., Ste. 481
Scottsdale, AZ 85251

Chapter 3

Biocompatible Dentistry

By Dr. S. David Buck and Dr. Paul G. Rubin

Many of you reading this book will be people who are greatly aware of health issues, particularly the improvement and maintenance of good health over a lifetime. As such, it is important to note that today—with the ever-increasing number of procedures, techniques, and modern equipment available—it is becoming increasingly evident that medicine must focus on problem-oriented practice. That is, medicine has become extremely specialized and proficient, and it is incumbent upon the practitioner to focus on a single problem and to solve **that** problem. As a result, the issue of whole-body medicine and maximizing health in a preventative sense—with a goal of increasing a person's quality of life—oftentimes is overlooked.

Dentistry typically has followed this outmoded, problem-oriented medical model. Evidence is growing that traditional dentistry, however well-intentioned, may have been contributing to generations of health problems. What has been overlooked has been attention to the whole person and concerns about how various dental materials may affect overall health. Biocompatible dentistry aims at optimal health for the whole individual. Materials and techniques are used that are *compatible* with health.

A great deal of concern has surfaced in the last several years about materials used in dentistry that may be *toxic* to the body.

Is there really cause for alarm? We believe there is—and that current scientific evidence supports this position. Chief among the offenders is the long-standard filling material, "silver" amalgam.

Amalgam is a mixture of silver, mercury, copper, and other trace metals used in dentistry for over 150 years. It is still the restorative material of choice for most U.S. dentists; in fact, a large portion of dentists worldwide still use mercury amalgam in their day-to-day practices.

There is now a tremendous body of scientific evidence that clearly and irrefutably has demonstrated that amalgam fillings, comprised of approximately 50% mercury, are, in fact, a source of toxic exposure to the body, as mercury vapor escapes from the fillings and enters the body quite readily.

We now know that elemental mercury is released in vapor form in very small amounts from fillings on an ongoing, daily basis. The amount of release is subject to some variation, based upon physical stimulation on the restorations, that is, chewing and hot/cold cycling. Chewing and hot/cold variations are a normal part of daily function, therefore, we can expect sustained minute release of mercury into the body in the form of mercury vapor throughout the life of the fillings.

The uptake of mercury into the body has been well established. Careful animal studies have demonstrated that mercury does, in fact, accumulate in the body. The nature of this exposure is long term and low grade. It is now suspected that many environmental toxins (i.e. lead, organic solvents, etc.) can have a deleterious effect on the body and on the overall state of health by virtue of a long-term, low-grade exposure mechanism. These other external environmental toxins have differing degrees of possibility of uptake into the body; silver/mercury amalgam, however, is implanted directly into the body, therefore, eliminating any opportunity to avoid detrimental exposure.

It has been estimated that the release of mercury into the body goes on year after year and will not stop until the filling itself falls out. There has been some evidence that when a silver/mercury filling is five years old, it is about 27% mercury, and that fillings 20 years old contain less than 5% mercury. So we know that the mercury is gone from the filling, but where does it go? If it comes off in the form of a vapor, the vapor will enter the lungs and be absorbed into the bloodstream. If it is incorporated into food while chewing, it will be swallowed, digested, and absorbed into the bloodstream. From the bloodstream, mercury has access to all parts of the body.

When one examines the scientific literature regarding the toxicity of mercury to humans, it is very clear that no safe level of mercury exposure has yet been determined. On the contrary, mercury is categorized as one of the most highly toxic metals known to man. Given the fact that mercury fillings release mercury into the body and that mercury is widely recognized as having significant toxic properties, one wonders why the organized profession of dentistry in the U.S. has not sought to restrict or eliminate its use.

The American Dental Association (ADA), a professional trade organization representing most United States dentists, still maintains that mercury amalgam is safe. However, they do so with no hard scientific data to back up their statements; their primary rationale for the continued use of amalgam is the fact that it has been used for so many years without massive epidemics of illness. This reasoning is flawed. As new advances in science occur, and we are allowed to look deeper into the hypotheses, naturally, we should reexamine our fundamental beliefs willingly in empirical scientific inquiry.

Fortunately, on an international level, dental amalgam is receiving a high degree of scrutiny. In Sweden, for instance, amalgam use is being curtailed and severely restricted; additionally, Germany now is looking at phasing out use of dental amalgam and already has recommended that it not be used in children and women of child-bearing age. Other countries, such as Japan and Australia, have reviewed basic scientific literature and decided to question heavily the use of amalgam. However, it still is held to be perfectly safe in both the United States and Canada, where it is used widely today.

How will this constant exposure to mercury affect one's health? Acute industrial levels of mercury exposure have identifiable symptoms. However, long-term, low-grade exposure doesn't necessarily result in the same pattern of symptoms as the acutely exposed patient; and no level of mercury exposure is considered healthy when you examine the various effects it has at the cellular level.

As a general overview of adverse health reactions, there are
five basic areas where there have been documented improvements,
once amalgam has been removed.

1. Neurological (or the nervous system), which really is divided
into two primary areas—the emotional and the motor. Depression,
irritability, and inability to cope are emotional problems which
have been noted to change dramatically upon amalgam removal.
Motor functions which result in seizures, muscle spasms, and
other types of illnesses also have responded positively.

2. Cardiovascular, which would be alterations of heart performance, such as unidentified chest pains or rapid heartbeat.

3. Collagen diseases—problems with the basic cementing
substances of the cells, such as arthritis, lupus, bursitis.

4. Immunological, which basically means how well your
immune system functions. Interference with this overall system
results in increased susceptibility to whatever illnesses are going
around.

5. Finally, allergies—mercury, in combination with the substance to which you are allergic, will rupture white blood cells
and can precipitate allergic reactions.

Another widely held belief is that there are no comparable
alternatives to the durability and strength of amalgam. As of
1995, that simply is not true. Properly placed, biocompatible
composites in teeth utilizing state-of-the-art equipment and
bonding techniques offer very good results that are very comparable to amalgam. Three- to five-year studies of composites
show extremely good results with respect to durability and wear.
So the two-fold argument—(1) that mercury amalgam is safe
and (2) that the alternatives to replacing amalgam are inferior—
simply is not true.

We want to emphasize that not every dental patient should
rush out immediately and have their amalgam fillings replaced.
First, that would be impossible because there are not enough
dental-care providers to accomplish this. Second, mercury—
although harmful—affects people differently. Some react in an
extremely minor way; those people probably can retain their
fillings with a minimal amount of damage. Other patients are
so sensitive that they experience severe reactions. We certainly
would recommend, however, that you never again let a dentist
place an amalgam filling in your mouth.

But what about the old fillings that are already there? If you make an informed decision to replace them, we urge you to work with someone who is experienced at this removal process. (Later, we will tell you how to find a properly trained dentist who can replace amalgam fillings safely and correctly.)

We would like to tell you about the pioneering work done by Dr. Hal Huggins of Colorado Springs, Colorado. Dr. Huggins has a multi-disciplinary treatment facility aimed at maximizing and increasing the health of patients with varying degrees of serious illness—not only through removal of mercury-containing amalgam, but through careful analysis of blood-chemistry values and balancing blood chemistry through various supplements, body disciplines, homeopathic remedies, and nutritional counseling. Dr. Huggins is one of the pioneers in exposing the mercury issue as it pertains to dental amalgam. Over many years, he has continued to teach, lecture, write, and treat patients, even under tremendous pressure from organized dental groups which have sought to suppress this vital information. Dr. Huggins undoubtedly has been responsible for changing the course of practice for hundreds of dentists across the United States, as well as internationally, who now practice a holistic form of dental care. So it is with great respect that we acknowledge the contributions of Dr. Huggins, as much of the information we are sharing in this book is a result of Dr. Huggins' work.

The History of the Use of Amalgam Fillings

Before about 160 years ago, in the early part of the 1800's, dentistry consisted mainly of restoring teeth with gold for those who could afford it...and a lot of extractions for those who couldn't! Then, two brothers came from Europe, bringing a new material that's not much different from what we still use as dental amalgam today, commonly known as "silver" dental fillings. It was a material that mixed fine filings of alloy of silver, copper, and zinc with liquid mercury, forming a paste which hardened in a few minutes. This revolutionized dentistry, in that teeth could be filled with a material that was relatively inexpensive and easy to use, which meant that a lot of people could have fillings placed who never before had been able to do so.

Many of the dentists at the time, however, were very concerned about this material, believing that it was not a good material

(not healthy) and that it shouldn't be used. Proponents of
amalgam fought a heavy battle; this was what we call the first
"amalgam war." The dentists who were against amalgam tried
to get dentists to sign an oath not to use this inferior material.
Although some did sign, the fact is that basically the strategy
didn't work; the economic pressures were too great for dentists
to have something affordable with which they could fill teeth
easily, thereby attracting more patients. A new society was formed
by those dentists who chose to use this amalgam material; that
new society was the forerunner of what today is called the
American Dental Association (ADA).

In the late 1970' and early '80's some concerns again came
to light, mainly through the efforts of Dr. Huggins who was
concerned that mercury from their fillings was affecting patients'
overall health. The word began to spread among a small number
of concerned dentists who were questioning the safety of amalgam. Then, in the early 1980's, some researchers began using
a sophisticated instrument which detected significant mercury
vapor levels in the mouths of people who had "silver" dental
fillings, and no mercury in the mouths of those who had no
amalgam fillings. Typically, the greater the number of fillings
in the mouth, the greater the amount of mercury vapor detected.
This proved to be conclusive evidence that mercury vapor does,
indeed, escape from "silver" dental fillings. At the same time,
this factor still was being denied by the ADA.

Throughout this time, there were also some preliminary studies
which seemed to point to a decreased immune capacity in the
presence of amalgam fillings in the mouth. By 1991, the World
Health Organization, after reviewing all the available research,
concluded that mercury from dental amalgams contributed the
greatest single source of mercury exposure in humans—greater
than food (including seafood) or the environment (including
various sources of air pollution). Still, even after this report came
out, the ADA was issuing statements such as: "You're going to
get more mercury from a tuna sandwich that you eat at lunch
today than from the dental fillings in your mouth." Clearly, this
is contrary to current scientific information.

Dentists generally have relied upon the ADA to provide them
with information and guidance. The ADA, unfortunately, has
been presenting a rather one-sided view, one that does not

correspond to the emerging evidence in the non-dental, scientific community. This has led some concerned dentists to work harder to seek out and sort out the mounting scientific evidence.

In 1984, an organization called The International Academy of Oral Medicine and Toxicology (IAOMT) was formed. This academy is dedicated to spreading information in the scientific community on the research being done with regard to issues of mercury and other topics of biocompatability in dentistry. This group also has been active in organizing and promoting research and, subsequently, has become one of the most authoritative bodies on the subject matter of mercury-free dentistry worldwide.

Some very sophisticated animal studies were designed in the early 1990's to examine the effects of dental amalgam mercury. This was done first by a research group at the University of Calgary Medical School, using pregnant sheep as a model. Amalgam fillings containing radioactive mercury were placed in a sheep's teeth. This enabled the researchers to trace the radio-active mercury through the body, knowing clearly that if they detected it somewhere other than the teeth, it could have come only from the "silver" fillings, as radioactive mercury does not exist anywhere in nature.

In a few days after placement of the amalgam fillings, radio-active mercury was detected in virtually all organs of the sheep's body. Within just a few weeks, it also was detectable in the fetal blood supply and in the fetal tissues. This accumulation in the fetal blood supply and tissues continued throughout the life of the fetus; in fact, the newborn got an additional dose of mercury through the mother's milk. This landmark study, published in a prestigious peer-reviewed scientific journal, caused quite a stir in the scientific community. It caused a bit of stir in the dental community, as well, but the response there was one of denial and criticism of the study.

Similar studies were repeated later in monkeys, with virtually the same results.

The Calgary research team also came out with information that not only did mercury accumulate in animal tissue, but they were able to demonstrate that the mercury was causing a 50% reduction in kidney function as well. A 50% reduction in kidney function doesn't mean kidney failure, nor does it necessarily mean an observable change in the health of the animal, but it would be the equivalent of walking around with only one kidney. This is a pathological change caused by mercury derived from silver amalgam fillings; it ought to be the "smoking gun" that puts an end to the use of amalgam fillings in dentistry. Yet, during this time period (just within the last few years), spokespeople from the ADA continue to deny that mercury is a problem, still maintaining that it is perfectly safe for use in human mouths.

Other studies performed at about the same time were done at the University of Georgia by a noted microbiologist. She discovered that bacteria normally living in the intestines became mercury resistant in the presence of mercury at levels equivalent to what one gets when exposed to mercury fillings. This became particularly significant when it was discovered that those mercury-resistant bacteria were becoming resistant to antibiotics, as well. So, there's a scenario where mercury from dental fillings in the mouth was creating an increase in antibiotic-resistant bacteria in the body. (Most of us are aware that the increase in antibiotic-resistant bacteria is becoming a real problem in medicine today, where it's becoming harder and harder to fight infections with antibiotics that are becoming more and more ineffective.)

There are studies under way at the University of Kentucky on the effect of mercury on brain tissue, particularly considering disorders such as Alzheimer's disease. Researchers have been finding, as recently as spring of 1995, that mercury creates a similar kind of neurological disarray that typically is found in Alzheimer's disease victims. As yet, they are not ready to come out and say that mercury causes Alzheimer's disease, but they are saying that mercury causes the same neurological change on a cellular level that is seen in Alzheimer's disease. This research is continuing.

A very recent study (within the last year or two of this writing) has linked mercury to effects discovered in dental office personnel. The study shows that dental assistants who work with amalgam have a 50% reduction in fertility. There is a correlation between fertility problems in female dental personnel who work with amalgam and the number of amalgam fillings per week that those assistants are handling. There is another recent study that was conducted on dentists, themselves, which shows the behavioral and psychomotor effects of mercury when comparing dentists with the general population. In April 1995, another paper in a prestigious peer-reviewed scientific journal discussed the issue of mercury exposure from "silver" tooth fillings, concluding that "research evidence does not support the notion of amalgam safety." So, the *scientific* community seems to be overwhemingly questioning the safety of dental amalgam.

Amalgam and the Environment

There's a related issue here on mercury and the environment. We know that mercury is toxic to humans. We also know that it is a significant environmental contaminant, and there are millions of dollars spent cleaning up toxic sites from industrial accidents that have spilled mercury. In addition, there is a great deal of effort made to control mercury emissions from industrial settings where mercury is used or potentially is expelled into the environment.

One industry that expels mercury into the environment which has been overlooked is dentistry! This began to come to light in this country a few years ago when some of the municipal organizations that handle waste treatment were beginning to see increased levels of mercury in the waste treatment facilities. In attempting to trace the mercury back to its point of origin, they began to discover that a significant amount of it was coming from dental offices. In Tucson, Seattle, San Francisco, and other cities where it has been studied, they are finding that somewhere between 14% and 25% of the mercury entering the waste treatment facilities comes from dental offices, a totally unregulated industry.

So, where does the mercury originate? Think back to your experiences in the dental chair when you had amalgam fillings placed or removed. Remember that little suction device which slurps up all of the saliva, water, and debris in the working area around the teeth? It's also slurping up any amalgam residue, amalgam scrap, and grindings from old amalgam fillings. Basically, all of that just goes down the drain. Dentists always have had little screens or traps that take out the big chunks, but there's a lot of amalgam sludge or slurry that goes right down the drain into the waste water system.

This has been a concern in European countries where they have stricter regulations on environmental emissions. Countries such as Sweden, Germany, and others, for a number of years have had regulations on dental offices, requiring them to place specific mercury filtration units in the offices to filter the water before it goes into the waste water system.

There never have been any such regulations in the United States, to this point. The concern over the last few years, however, may be leading to that. For instance, the greater Seattle area came very close to passing a regulation in 1994 which would have required filtration units to be installed in all dental offices. This since has been changed to a "strong recommendation," but not yet a requirement. Other cities are beginning to come to the same conclusion...that this is a significant problem.

It is potentially a problem to the waste treatment facilities because they often take the sludge—or what is called "biosolids" —that is left over from treatment of waste water and sell it to be used as fertilizer on farms and forest lands. In some areas of the country, the material is incinerated. There are EPA regulations on how much heavy metal can be in this material; and if there's too much mercury in it, then the municipality can't sell it, can't call it fertilizer, and may be regulated with regard to incineration (which, of course, would send vapors of heavy metal right into the atmosphere).

We are very proud to say that in our office we do have a mercury filtration system. We have had it for several years, and we were one of the first in the country to have had one installed. Still, we're just one of a handful of dentists who have taken responsible action on our own to do our part in cleaning up the environment by not allowing mercury waste material to enter the waste water system. Predictably, the ADA has denied that this is a problem and vigorously fought any regulations to require such units in all dental offices.

There is likely to be more information and more publicity about the mercury-in-the-environment issue in the coming years. In fact, it was the environmental issue that finally was the last straw that caused the Swedish Parliament to pass regulations actually phasing out entirely the use of amalgam in their country over the next couple of years. Similar concerns by the Ministry of the Environment and Energy in the province of Ontario, Canada (April, 1995) may have a serious impact on future amalgam use in Ontario.

Other Issues in the Practice of Holistic Dentistry

Other than the obvious area of mercury amalgam, there are other important considerations for a patient preparing to undergo removal of mercury-based amalgam. One of these is the issue of root-canal teeth. This is another deeply controversial area in dentistry today. Concern has been resurfacing, based on research done in the early 1900's by Dr. Weston Price, that there may be problems with teeth that have been treated with root-canal fillings. Some dentists and physicians hold to the theory that root-canal-treated teeth—even ones that have no symptoms and look perfectly "normal" on X-rays—still may harbor bacteria in the porosities of the root structure. It is believed that these bacteria are capable of producing harmful bacterial toxins that can enter the bloodstream and contribute to a variety of degenerative health problems in other parts of the body. Some believe that these teeth should be extracted, as they pose too much of a potential hazard to health.

This is a very difficult decision to make, and it is an area where more research needs to be done. We don't presume to have a clear, black-and-white answer here, but we do want you to know about this issue, read available information (we'd recommend *Root Canal Coverup Exposed,* by George Meinig, DDS, Bion Publishing), and discuss it with your dentist.

Another area gaining the attention of holistic-oriented dentists is what is known as a jawbone cavitation. As the name implies, these are holes in the jawbone where healthy bone structure is missing. In the medical literature, they are being referred to as NICO (neuralgia inducing cavitational osteonecrosis) lesions. Authors in several studies have reported that once these cavitational lesions are surgically removed, a tremendous decrease in pain symptoms often is achieved. These lesions seem to happen as an aftereffect of some tooth extractions. They are very hard to detect on X-rays, so they often are overlooked. Based upon laboratory findings, one or more of the following factors can contribute to a NICO lesion developing after an extraction: immune system dysfunction or deficiency, the presence of unusual microbial pathogens, reduced blood flow to the affected area, a lack of one or more bone growth factors being present, and nerve dysfunction.

Many dentists, now armed with this new knowledge, alter the normal routine in which they take out teeth, particularly in extracting root-canal teeth or wisdom teeth. Special techniques are used in order to avoid developing such cavitations. These areas, when identified, can be eliminated successfully with a relatively simple oral surgical procedure. As with the root-canal issue, the traditional view that "normal-appearing X-rays and lack of symptoms means everything is healthy" just isn't enough. We must look further at the effects that we, as dentists, are creating on overall health, and we feel that you need to be adequately informed to discuss these issues with your dentist (who, unfortunately, also may not be informed thoroughly).

Another important area to discuss is the interaction of other materials used in dentistry on the body's immune system. Again, through the pioneering work of Dr. Huggins, it has been discovered (through complex immune testing) that the immune system can be quite reactive to many of the materials and agents used in routine, everyday dental practice. Most notable of these are other metals used to fabricate various appliances, crowns, bridgework, and even dentures.

Unfortunately, one of the more unrecognized, but potentially harmful metals routinely used in dentistry today, is nickel. Many porcelain crowns have been placed on teeth to make them look like natural teeth, but the porcelain was fused to a non-precious alloy that is nickel based. Nickel apparently has a high degree of immune reactivity in many patients and appears to be one of the highest potential aggravators to the immune system.

Clinical Protocol in Our Office for Treating Mercury-Removal Patients

What does all this mean in "real people" terms? What effect does all of this have on patients? What kinds of things do we do in our office? This brings us to the importance of how we treat the patient from start to finish in our office, with regard to holistic dental practice and improving a patient's health.

The first thing we do is encourage patients to undergo a dental-materials compatibility test, which seeks to confirm which dental materials have the lowest immune reactivity to the patient's own blood serum. Then, by choosing materials with the least allergic or adverse-reaction potential and by placing only *those* materials in the patient's mouth, we feel we're providing the best care we possibly can.

After compatability testing, patients are encouraged to seek care with a physician (M.D. or naturopathic) who will work closely with our office. The holistic physician provides overall counseling and testing, ascertaining deficiencies the patient may have in his/her own individual metabolism. By seeking not only to balance these deficiencies, but to provide protective and detox supplementation, the patient is maximally protected.

What we mean when we say "detox" is that there are certain agents, techniques, and procedures that will help the body to rid itself of heavy metals. The agents bind to the mercury and assist in excreting it from the body's tissues, as mercury is stored in varying amounts in various places in the body. Simply removing it from the mouth eliminates the highest source of exposure, but the body still may be dealing with a load of heavy metal that needs to be pulled out and excreted.

It is also important to note that patients who are seeking improvement in overall health will gain substantially by supplementing and/or altering their diets, as well as following the medical advice of the physician, as it pertains to the results revealed by the physical and laboratory reports.

For example, a large portion of our patient group falls into the category of symptomology we call "chronic fatigue." These patients have varying symptoms, with the common threads being a lack of energy, poor sleeping patterns, changes in appetite, changes in ability to concentrate, and a decrease in overall energy from a prior time. Such patients benefit maximally from the services and care of a holistic physician, in conjunction with mercury removal. We see dramatic improvements in these patients' energy levels, and they report to us feeling much better about their own health.

After a patient has obtained compatibility testing and has begun the process of blood-chemistry balancing through working with a physician, we then can begin the actual amalgam removal, which is done in a specialized sequence and with careful attention to scheduling appointments so as not to unduly stress the immune system. Typically, the teeth are restored in "quadrants" (one-fourth of the mouth at a time), and appointments usually take from 1½ to 2 hours.

Finally, when the patient is being treated, there are certain clinical protocols which maximize protection for the patient and minimize exposure to mercury vapor. Our dental treatment facility provides for two levels of protection for patients. Those who are quite symptomatic and require maximum protection from mercury vapor can be treated in rooms which have negative ion generators. These rooms have the cleanest air supply and the least possibility of generating or retaining mercury vapor of any amount in the air. Additionally, all patients receive treatment under a rubber dam. Patients also will breathe oxygen through a nose mask, which minimizes breathing air in the vicinity during amalgam removal. In addition, we use copious irrigation during the actual drilling sequence; heavy water flow and high-volume suction are used to create a minimum of vapor when removing mercury-based amalgam. Patients also are covered fully with protective drapes, and protective eye gear is worn.

After amalgam removal is complete and the dental revision has been accomplished, patients will follow up with the physician to continue detoxification through chelation to remove heavy metals, as well as dietary review, supplementation, and possibly homeopathic remedies to bring the body back into balance and increase immune function and energy levels.

How to Find a Dentist Utilizing Biocompatible Techniques

The dentists across the country practicing biocompatible dentistry are relatively small in number, but they tend to network with each other. There are also a couple of organizations that have lists and referral services to help find a suitable, mercury-free, biocompatible dentist in or near your area. One such organization is the Huggins Diagnostic Clinic in Colorado Springs, which has a toll-free telephone number (1-800-331-2303). The other organization is called Foundation for Toxic-Free Dentistry (FTFD), which provides information on mercury-free dentistry and a referral list to someone in your area, if you write to them and include a self-addressed stamped envelope: The Foundation for Toxic-Free Dentistry, P. O. Box 608010, Orlando, FL 32860-8010.

We recommend interviewing a prospective dental office by asking the following questions to help determine if this is the office for you:

1. How do they feel about mercury amalgam fillings? Comment: If the dentist says something like, "Well, we don't really feel that that's a problem; but if you want a non-mercury filling, we'll go ahead and put one in for you," I'd be leery of their level of commitment.

2. Have they had any specialized education and training in mercury-free dentistry? Two organizations that are providing training and experience in all the issues surrounding mercury-free dentistry are The International Academy of Oral Medicine and Toxicology (IAOMT) and the Huggins Diagnostic Clinic. Training and experience are crucial to doing this type of dentistry safely and effectively for patients.

3. Are they committed to a mercury-free practice? Does the dentist still sometimes place amalgam, if requested, or does he/she still feel there are places where amalgams are appropriate? Comment: I would question his/her level of commitment to taking the necessary precautionary steps in replacing amalgam fillings safely.

4. Do they have amalgam fillings in their own mouths? Comment: Have they put their commitment where their mouth is?

5. Do they work with other health practitioners who can advise on mercury detoxification, nutrition, balancing body chemistry, etc.? This is an extremely important part of proper care in replacement of amalgam fillings with respect to overall dental and general health.

For the potential patient seeking to remove mercury-based amalgam fillings, it is important to ask your dentist good questions and become informed. It is your body, and you have the right to know.

We also feel it is important to find a dentist who is familiar with placing non-amalgam fillings, particularly in posterior teeth. Although all dentists are trained to use composite materials, the placement of composite and non-mercury-based materials in posterior teeth requires great attention to detail. Poor technique and inattention to detail will result in a marginally acceptable treatment result, likely to have a short life of service. One can expect a very durable and long life of service from non-amalgam posterior composite fillings from a dentist who is comfortable with and frequently places posterior composites and uses state-of-the-art materials and techniques.

Additionally, the dentist should be comfortable in interpreting compatibility reports and understanding the need for compatibility testing. Patient protective measures, at minimum, should include rubber dams, additional irrigation, and high-volume suction to remove mercury-based fillings.

Finally, your dentist should be aware of and be able to answer questions regarding root-canal teeth and cavitations. These adjunctive areas are particularly important for the patient who is not well systemically. An otherwise healthy patient still may benefit from the removal of mercury-based amalgam fillings; however, the patient who already is compromised needs additional protective measures, as well as consideration for the adjunctive areas of treatment to maximize recovery.

S. David Buck, D.D.S., P.S. and Paul G. Rubin, D.D.S.

Dr. S. David Buck graduated from the University of Washington School of Dentistry in 1988. He has been committed to continuing education in dentistry and recently has attended advance training at the Huggins Diagnostic Center. Dr. Buck is also a member of the International Academy of Oral Medicine and Toxicology. He is active in local business and civic groups in the Seattle area.

Dr. Paul G. Rubin graduated from The University of Washington School of Dentistry in 1973. He has been practicing mercury-free dentistry since 1981. He is a past president of the Washington Society for Preventive Dentistry and is a Fellow of the International Academy of Oral Medicine and Toxicology. Dr. Rubin has lectured and done research on topics related to mercury toxicity and dentistry.

Dr. Buck and Dr. Rubin practice at the Broadway Dental Center, 310 Harvard Avenue East, Seattle, WA 98102; their telephone number is (206) 324-1100.

Chapter 4

Nature's Nutrition

By Dr. Tom Corbitt and Dr. Dee Corbitt

The American public has been brainwashed into thinking they are going to die from some disabling disease such as cancer, heart disease, arthritis, high blood pressure, diabetes, etc. Dr. Tom Corbitt and Dr. Dee Corbitt, founders of Nature's Nutrition, have written the following information to let *you* know *You Can LIVE!* Yes, you can live and have vibrant health for a lifetime. Imagine this: You can determine how long you live! You can control your own health! This information is provided so that *you* can be informed about the latest scientific, medical, and nutritional information on such organic nutritional supplements as:

The Capsule—the only organic nutritional supplement available anywhere which contains *all* 18 elements necessary to sustain the human body.

Cat's Claw—a Peruvian herb beneficial in the treatment of cancer, arthritis, bursitis, rheumatism, genital herpes and herpes zoster, allergies, ulcers, systemic candidiasis, PMS and other female problems, environmental toxin poisoning, many bowel and intestinal disorders, organic depression, and those infected with the HIV virus.

O.E.F.—Oscillating Energy Factors and Pycnogenol with pro-anthocyanidins from the grape pips—absolutely imperative for the defusing of free radicals before they form in the body.

Herbal Formulas—over 55 nutritional herbal formula combinations to help put the body chemistry in balance so the body can heal itself.

The Capsule

"The Capsule" is the most exciting natural organic nutritional supplement ever developed. There never before has been a natural organic food and herb supplement that contains every nutrient the body requires...but now you have it in "The Capsule." The first thing we must understand about nutrition is that God made our bodies to receive the nutrients (vitamins, minerals, amino acids, proteins, calcium, live enzymes, etc.) from the food that we eat. All of the nutrients in The Capsule are in their natural organic form and have not been altered by man, so the body can assimilate them easily.

Hippocrates, the father of all medicine, said, "Let your food be your medicine and your medicine be your food."

Nutritionists today believe that philosophy and seek to help people build their good health with natural sources. Herbs such as Green Barley, Ginseng, Pollen, etc., are considered to be food rather than medicine because they are complete, all natural, and pure—as nature intended. When these herbs are taken, the body starts to be cleansed, purifying itself. This gives the body nutrients to function as God intended. Unlike chemically-synthesized, highly-concentrated, so-called vitamins and drugs that produce countless side effects, herbs can realign the body's defenses, helping it to heal itself without any side effects.

At the dawn of creation, the whole world was covered with plant life, endless variety and beauty—from the lowest form of plant life (algae) growing in water, to the highest and most completely developed plants, such as grass. Alongside this flora existed animal life, from the simplest amoeba to the highest and most complete of God's creations—Man.

Let us reflect for a few minutes on what this means. It means that living creatures, including man, have been fed and sustained by herbs, and by herbs alone. For if we eat the flesh of animals, we are but eating chewed and digested grasses. If we drink milk or eat butter, it is the same thing; namely chewed grass. However, in such cases we get the vital nutrients (or life principal) second hand (diminished from its original state) because much of the life has been used by the animal who ate it first, and whose flesh we subsequently eat. This is a good argument for the vegetarian and a strong point in their favor. Also, whenever you cut through the flesh of any animal, you have as much veinous blood as arterial blood. And the veinous blood contains the waste matter and debris of that animal's cells. Another vegetarian argument is that animal flesh is subject to putrefaction and produces very poisonous alkaloids, while vegetables in the process of decay do not produce putrefaction or alkaloids.

All life on earth always has been dependent upon this vegetable or herb kingdom. This is true now and will continue to be true as long as there is life on the earth. However, we must understand that our lives and health do not depend upon the foods we eat, but upon the nutrition our bodies derive from those foods. If we eat food of little or no nutritional value, our immune system becomes depleted and sickness and disease begin. Vitamin manufacturers give the impression in their advertising that vitamins will increase energy and help ward off sickness. The fact is that vitamins in themselves do not give us energy or make us feel good; their value is in their ability to make the carbohydrates, fats, and proteins in our diets available for use as energy. By themselves, they cannot cure anything. The food factors must be present for energy and cell regeneration.

Americans are buying vitamins at a rate in excess of $2 billion a year. Yet, there is still much doubt whether these synthetic substitutes can replace the real nutrients found in foods. Critics warn that the uninformed who use vitamins do so at their own peril, and they cite many cases of overdose and vitamin toxicity. On the other hand, we know the nutrients found in food are safe and can sustain good health.

Let's consider the content of The Capsule. We start with what is considered to be the most nutritious plant on earth, green barley. It contains all of your vitamins, minerals, amino acids, enzymes, fiber (soluble and non-soluble), chlorophyll, calcium, and complete proteins. It is richer in calcium than ordinary milk or dairy foods. It is richer in iron than many foods like spinach, and it is abundant in potassium and magnesium. Its vitamins and minerals activate enzymes which are known to be the spark of life. It supplies in balance the full spectrum of the B-complex vitamin family—more effective proteins than will be found in meat or milk source. One of the important enzymes is S.O.D.

(Super-oxide Dismutase), which protects cells against free
radicals. Dr. Schnable, chemist and plant scientist, stated that
there are nutrients in whole leaf green barley that science has
yet to discover. To get all these nutrients, it must be organically-
grown, whole-leaf barley, not a dried-juice barley.

The next food in The Capsule is bee pollen. Dr. Pavo Airola,
long considered America's foremost nutritionist and a leading
world authority on holistic health and biological medicine, states
multisource bee pollen is the richest and most complete food
in nature. It increases the body's resistance to stress and disease
and speeds up the healing process in most conditions of ill health.
Bee pollen also possesses age-retarding and rejuvenating properties. One of the most beneficial effects of bee pollen is that it
quickly produces the same anti-putrefaction effect as lactic acid
foods, thus contributing to a healthy digestive system and good
assimilation of nutrients—absolute prerequisites for good health
and long life. Bee pollen truly is a miracle food, wonder medicine,
and fountain of youth.

Next in The Capsule is royal jelly, which provides sustained
high energy, invigorating vitality, improved mental alertness, and
stamina. It is one of the world's richest natural sources of pantothenic acid, which has been called the antistress nutrient. This
nutrient is believed to combat stress, fatigue, and insomnia, and
is essential for healthy skin and hair. Royal jelly also contains
all eight of the essential amino acids, as well as the minerals
calcium, iron, potassium, and silicon. Royal jelly has worldwide
credibility. In Japan it is the nation's best-selling supplement.
In England, members of the Royal family, including Princess
Diana, use it. In China, the passion for royal jelly is legendary,
as millions praise its immediate and long-lasting benefits.

Next in The Capsule we have gotu kola, an Indian herb that
acts to strengthen and revitalize worn out bodies and brain cells,
thus preventing brain fatigue. Known as the secret to perpetual
youth, it strengthens the heart, memory, and brain. It helps
hormone balance—a truly necessary and wonderful herb.

Next in The Capsule is Siberian ginseng, known for its value
for thousands of years. It possesses a wide range of therapeutic
activity, increases sexual health in men and women, and builds
zest, energy, stamina, and endurance. Siberian ginseng also
increases mental and physical work ability, helps combat everyday

weariness, and improves mental and physical reflex action. It protects the body against stress and produces a strengthening effect.

The final herb in The Capsule is Thalophyte. Thalophyte is a remarkable nutrient that provides the human body with what we loosely call vitamins, in the form of chlorides, iodides, bromides, phosphates, and sulfates of calcium, magnesium, potassium, and sodium. All of them are positive organic salts absolutely necessary to the healthy metabolism of the human body.

In the preceding paragraph, I mentioned nutrients loosely called vitamins. The reason I said that is because there is no such thing as Vitamins A, B, C, D, E, or any other letter in the alphabet. They do not exist except in the imagination of unscientific minds, who first originated the idea, or those who believe it because it is advertised so heavily. The word *vita* means "to live." The word *min* is an abbreviation of the Latin word *minimus*, which is "the smallest drop of liquid." Therefore, a vitamin is "the tiniest drop of liquid life."

No one ever has defined the word *life*, and they also have not shown its chemical composition, because life is not capable of being weighed. It is not solid, liquid, nor gaseous, and it is beyond man's wisdom to define.

The word vitamin probably was intended to convey the idea that certain substances are cell foods that vitalize organs and cells of the human body. Since we know what these substances are and have an extensive knowledge of them and of their chemical constitution, we need to stop using senseless terminology—such as "vitamins"—and find out how these vitalizing substances can be used to promote more life and vigor to our body.

About 150 years ago a group of scientists from around the world made an intensive study of the chemistry of the human body, chemically analyzing the particular organs, tissues, and parts of the body; they found that the entire human body is comprised of only 18 elements. The findings of these devoted scientists are as follows: (1) the structure of the human body is built and vitalized by calcium phosphate, calcium carbonate, and magnesium phosphate, (2) the brain and nerves by potassium and magnesium phosphate, (3) connective tissue cells by silica, (4) muscular tissues by magnesium, potassium, and calcium phosphates and chlorides, (5) elastic tissues by calcium fluoride, (6) blood by iron phosphate, etc. It is important to have some knowledge of what makes up your body, because every disease known to man is primarily a condition of unbalanced chemistry of both elements and compounds which compose the tissues and fluids of the body.

Thalophyte's phosphates of calcium, potassium, sodium, and magnesium, feed the bones, brain, liver, and flesh, respectively. Its potassium chloride dissolves fibrin, relieving inflammation of the mucous membrane, while its sodium chloride regulates the necessary amount of water in the system (which we know is the great ionizer and producer of vital chemical changes in the fluids of the body). Finally, its magnesium phosphate supplies material for the nourishment of muscle. When we finish, we will have covered five-sixths of all requirements of the body, so far as physical substance is concerned.

There is such an immense amount of subject matter concerning this herb that volumes could be written without exhausting it. Its chemistry reveals that it is strongly alkaline, and that its alkalinity is not dependent upon bicarbonate of soda, potash, or citric acid, like the much-advertised alkalizers. Alkalizers only serve the purpose of temporary relief of acid stomach, and if they get into the blood, they destroy its hemoglobin. Thalophyte, on the other hand, presents every cell in the body with sweet organic alkaline salts of four out of seven metals which nature uses to build and vitalize the human body. It does not lower or devitalize. On the contrary, it purifies, strengthens, and vitalizes nearly nine-tenths of the cellular structure and vital fluids of the body. Let us look a little closer into its chemistry to determine the reasons. It is well known that the thyroid and other glands require minute quantities of iodine for healthy function. Thalophyte supplies just such minute quantities in the form of sodium and potassium iodides. For some incredible reason, this mere trace of iodine works wonders on the glandular system, often changing the whole chemistry from disease to health.

Again, that mysterious element fluorine unites with the metal calcium to form calcium fluoride. This is found in the surface of bone, the enamel of teeth, the walls of blood vessels, and in all connective tissues and elastic fiber. The tensile strength, resiliency, and elasticity of the muscular system, the vascular system, the lymphatic system, the osseous system, and the connective tissues of the nervous system all largely depend upon relatively minute quantities of calcium fluoride—just a fractional part of the whole, but absolutely necessary, nevertheless. When there is the least shortage of calcium fluoride, a long series of disastrous effects are started. If the shortage occurs in the periosteum, periostitis sets in (nature is trying to supply the deficiency). The next state is periosteomyelitis. Usually, this results in abnormal bone growth, periosteophyma. When the shortage occurs in the enamel of teeth, decay quickly results. If in the vascular system, a very large number of so-called diseases arise which would take months to describe. A few examples will suffice: enlarged and flaccid heart, aneurysm, varicose veins, veinules, capillaries, etc., apoplexy, hemorrhage of the lungs or any other part, relaxation of the abdominal walls, with sagging of the whole abdominal walls, with sagging of the whole abdominal viscera, prolapsed uterus and anus, flaccidity of the whole muscular system, chronic wrinkling of the skin, particularly of the face and neck, indurated glands, lumpy exudations and growths on the surface of bones, encysted tumors, hard swelling, great weakness, and hundreds of other dreadful conditions too numerous to mention.

Just as a rose collapses without sufficient water, so will bone collapse without sufficient calcium phosphate; blood without sufficient iron; brain without sufficient potassium phosphate; heart without sufficient calcium chloride. All cells will decay and produce pus without sufficient sulfur. The lungs will collapse without enough oxygen. The hair will die without silica. The glands will cease to function without iodine. The skin tissues throughout the whole system will atrophy and die without calcium fluoride.

No one ever should be without The Capsule and the vital nutrients it provides. Now you can understand why all other so-called vitamin supplements are obsolete.

Nature's Nutrition is excited to be able to bring you such a wonderful product for your good health. *Nature* is ever young and beautiful, ever vibrant with life and more life, *why not man?* To obtain The Capsule, just call our toll-free number:

1-800-242-1115

GOOD HEALTH TO YOU!

Haridra

Haridra is the most effective antioxidant and free-radical scavenging herb in existence. The aging process exemplifies the cumulative result of deterioration of individual cells, tissues, and organs caused and promoted by free radicals. These mechanisms are known as the body's antioxidant defense reaction. Unfortunately, in most cases, the antioxidant defense is gradually overwhelmed by the aging process, or a disease, or both. The inflammatory processes associated with microbial or viral infections and the progression of cancer are just a few disease conditions which contribute to depletion of the antioxidant defense system of the body. Therefore it is of great importance to preserve the body's defenses against damages by free radicals.

Haridra curcuminoids are natural phenolic compounds with potent antioxidant properties. Several research groups and studies recently have provided convincing evidence as to how great the antioxidant properties of Haridra actually are.

The properties of the curcuminoids in Haridra in preventing build-up of tissue-injuring free radicals, particularly those responsible for the cardiovascular disease lipid peroxides, are among the better-known antioxidant properties of these compounds. The curcuminoids in Haridra were shown to prevent lipid peroxides formation in a much higher degree than the pycnogenol with pine bark extract, grape seed extract, or a synthetic antioxidant like B.H.T., which has shown to be toxic. The results of these experiments are indicated in the graph below.

The effect of Haridra curcuminoids used in the experiment is known as C-3 Complex and is the most effective antioxidant known. The study used volunteers to evaluate the antioxidant property of Haridra in preventing serum lipid peroxidation. Administration of Haridra resulted in a significant reduction of lipid peroxides formation and a decrease in the level of total cholesterol. These results clearly illustrate the potential role of Haridra in the prevention and treatment of heart disease.

The nutritional role of Haridra extract as anticarcinogenic (preventing the development of cancer) and antimutagenic (preventing damage to genetic material DNA) has been the subject of recent research.

Cancer-causing agents (carcinogens) belong to a diversified

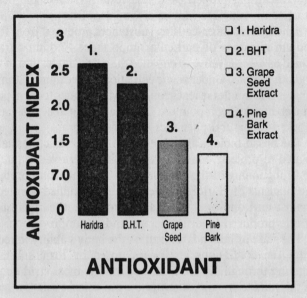

The effectiveness of Haridra is evident.

group of chemicals, originating from food, food contaminants, food additives, food-processing agents, environmental pollutants, synthetic chemicals, pharmaceutical drugs, and cosmetics. The development of cancer is a multistep process involving many factors, rather than a single one. Cancer-causing agents either can initiate tumors, promote tumors, or act as complete carcinogens, having both tumor-initiating and promoting activity. Likewise, cancer-preventing agents may prevent tumor initiation or promotion stages in tumor development.

Haridra extracts have been found to be cancer-preventing compounds in different tumor models, as well as in limited human studies.

The nutritional quality of food is known to change with cooking. For example, when cooking at high temperature, amino acids undergo a chemical change called pyrolysis. As a result, they may be converted into compounds with cancer-causing properties. Haridra curcuminoids inhibit the formation of these cancer-causing properties. These results validate the healthy practice of using Haridra as a food supplement.

Among the cancer-causing substances produced from foods, sodium nitrate is of particular importance. Sodium nitrate is added as a preservative to enhance the color and texture of meat and other foods. Under acidic conditions in the human stomach, amines and amides react chemically with nitrates to form potent cancer-causing compounds. This damaging reaction can be blocked by natural phenolics such as Haridra.

The broad biological activity of Haridra extract basically is related to protective mechanisms, which preserve the integrity and functioning of the human body. Two important protective mechanisms of Haridra extract have been studied—protection against environmental pollutants and protection against side effects produced by drug therapy and chemoprevention.

The state of health is a result of the body's ability to recover from the continuous challenges posed by toxic substances entering through air, food, and water. The most vivid example of this minute-by-minute struggle is our defense reaction against chemicals that cause cancer.

Haridra also has been evaluated in the treatment of inflammation associated with various forms of arthritis. The antiarthritic properties of Haridra were tested in a double-blind clinical trial in 49 patients with diagnosed rheumatoid arthritis. Haridra administered at a dose of 1200 mg per day for five to six weeks produced significant improvement in all patients. All patients showed overall improvement in morning stiffness and physical endurance.

Haridra also was used to treat patients with chronic respiratory disorders, with resulting subjective improvement of the condition and significant relief in symptoms like cough and labored breathing.

In view of the recently discovered applications, the properties of Haridra can be summarized best as protective properties. The protective quality of Haridra translates into the results of current research which prove that Haridra protects the integrity of biomolecules in the body. Haridra exerts a role in the body by protecting living tissue from being exposed to degenerative processes. Clinical and laboratory research indicate that diets supplemented with Haridra stabilize and protect biomolecules in the body at the molecular level. Haridra and its active principle, the curcuminoids, can exert protection either directly, by shielding the biomolecule, or indirectly, by stimulating the natural detoxification and defense mechanisms of the body.

I urge everyone to take the nutritional supplement Haridra on a daily basis and to make it available to everyone you know. Protection from the lifestyle diseases, i.e., cancer, heart disease, arthritis, premature aging, etc., is of the utmost importance.

Cat's Claw

This information is about a remarkable and exciting new herb from the rain forest in Peru. It is called *Uncaria tomentosa,* commonly known as Cat's Claw in English. For the purpose of this writing, we will be referring to this exceptional herb as Cat's Claw. The following facts appeared in the Townsend Letter for Doctors #130, May 1994.

Cat's Claw is an herb that grows wild in the highlands of the Peruvian Amazon. It has been used for hundreds, perhaps thousands, of years by native Indians for treatment of a wide range of health problems associated with the immune and digestive systems.

Starting in the early 1970's and continuing through today, research on this amazing plant has been conducted in many institutions throughout the world. Included in these prestigious institutions are the University of Milan and Naples, Italy; the University of Munich, Germany; the University of Innsbruck, Austria; The Huntington Research Center, England, and many other research facilities. The result of this research is that there is evidence that Cat's Claw may be beneficial in the treatment of cancer, arthritis, bursitis, rheumatism, genital herpes and herpes zoster, allergies, ulcers, systemic candidiasis, PMS and other female problems, environmental toxin poisoning, many bowel and intestinal disorders, organic depression, and those infected with the HIV virus.

Dr. Brent Davis, who has been working with Cat's Claw in the United States for a number of years, has referred to this herb as "The Opener of the Way" because of its remarkable ability to cleanse the entire intestinal tract and help patients suffering from many different stomach and bowel disorders, including: Crohn's disease, leaky bowel syndrome, diverticulitis, colitis, hemorrhoids, fistulas, gastritis, ulcers, parasites, and intestinal flora imbalance. In its healing ability and benefit to the immune system, Cat's Claw has so many therapeutic applications that it far surpasses such well-known herbs as Pau de Arco, Echinacea, Golden Seal, Astragulas, and Siberian Ginseng, as well as Reishi and Shitake Mushrooms and other products such as Citrus Seed Extract, Caprylic Acid, and Shark Cartilage.

In 1988, at the International Congress of Traditional Medicines in Lima, Peru, Cat's Claw was discussed by medical doctors as one of a number of different herbs used to consistently cure cancer and other serious disorders. One Peruvian physician spoke about his and his colleagues' successes with Cat's Claw and other herbs in treating 14 types of accurately diagnosed cancer in 700 patients between 1984 and 1988.

In an article by Dr. Davis, "A New World Class Herb," he talks about Cat's Claw's ability to break through severe intestinal derangements that no other available product can touch. He comes to this conclusion after treating approximately 150 patients from 1988 until 1992.

In July of 1989, a U.S. Patent was issued to a Dr. Klaus Keplinger, an Austrian research scientist, for isolating six oxindole alkaloids from the root of Cat's Claw. In this ten-page technical patent, it states that all but two of these alkaloids are suitable for the unspecific stimulating of the immunologic system. The most immunologically active alkaloid, according to the patent, is Isopteropodine. Isopteropodine (Isomer A), and to a lesser extent three of the other alkaloids, have been shown in laboratory testing to leave a pronounced enhancement effect on phago-cytosis (the ability of the white blood cells and macrophages to attack, engulf, and digest harmful microorganisms, foreign matter, and debris).

Research conducted at the Shanghai College of Traditional Chinese Medicine, shows that one of the remaining two alkaloids that does not have immune-stimulating properties, has been shown in laboratory testing to display an ability to inhibit platelet aggregation and thrombosis. This suggests that this alkaloid may be useful in the prevention of stroke and reducing the risk of heart attack by lowering blood pressure, increasing circulation, and inhibiting both the formation of plaque on the arterial walls and the formation of blood clots in the vessels of the brain, heart, and arteries.

On November 28, 1988, and June 17, 1993, articles about Cat's Claw appeared in *El Comercio*, the major metropolitan newspaper in Lima, Peru. The first article stated that Cat's Claw has been proven effective in the treatment of allergies and Neuro-bronchitis. The article then went on to talk about Dr. Keplinger's success in using Cat's Claw to treat genital herpes and herpes zoster. It ended with a discussion of his results in treating seven AIDS patients who displayed various progressions of the disease. According to the article, he was not able to help two of these patients. However, the well-being of the other five improved to such an extent that their symptoms disappeared.

The second article spoke about how Immodal, a laboratory in Austria under the direction of Dr. Keplinger, is using a medicine extracted from the vine of Cat's Claw along with AZT. This combination is being used to impede the multiplication of the HIV virus in the blood, activate the cells of the immune system, and stop the development of cancerous cells. The article went on to state that Immodal has commercialized this medicine under the name Krallendorn and has been using it successfully for the past six years to treat people infected with the AIDS virus. According to Immodal, practically none of the cases not yet showing symptoms of the disease developed further. The cases that displayed the first symptoms of the disease showed an improvement in blood analysis and a disappearance of clinical symptoms within the first year, a situation that continues to this day. Finally, the article mentioned that Krallendorn also has been effective in decreasing the unpleasant side effects of both AZT and radiation therapy when used in cancer treatment.

Besides Isopteropodine and other oxindole alkaloids, Italian and Peruvian researchers have isolated other beneficial items inherent in Cat's Claw, including several polyphenols, triterpines, and the plant steroids Beta-sitosterol, stigmasterol, and campesterol. The presence of these additional compounds might further explain Cat's Claw's antioxidant properties, its ability to protect cells from damage caused by free radicals, and the antiviral, antitumor, and anti-inflammatory properties also attributed to this herb.

In Peru and other Spanish-speaking countries, the common name for *Uncaria tomentosa* is Una de Gato—in English, Cat's

Claw. It is important to note that there is another *Uncaria* species
that grows in the lowlands of the Peruvian rain forests known
as *Uncaria guianensis*. This herb also is called Una de Gato and
Cat's Claw.

Uncaria guianensis has been shown to have some of the same
characteristics as *Uncaria tomentosa,* with one major exception.
Guianensis does not contain the most important alkaloid,
Isopteropodine. This would cause the species to be less effective
for the immune system applications. It is, therefore, important
to know that products being marketed as Cat's Claw can be either
Uncaria guianensis or *Uncaria tomentosa.*

In the highly acclaimed, best-selling book *Vibrational Healing*
by Dr. Richard Gerber, MD, Cat's Claw is mentioned as a unique
herbal remedy that has been used for many years by native
healers of Peru. He further states that the herb shows great
promise for the treatment of arthritis, when taken internally,
either by making a tea or taking capsules of the herb. Dr. Gerber
also explains that European studies have determined that Cat's
Claw has very low toxicity level, even if taken in large quantities
by those individuals who suffer from painful joints and cannot
take conventional medicines because of unpleasant side effects.
Finally, he suggests that Cat's Claw might be helpful in reducing
the side effects of radiation and chemotherapy associated with
cancer treatments.

Dr. Brent Davis says, "Cat's Claw is a world-class herb which
has the power to arrest and reverse deep-seated pathology,
allowing a more rapid return to health...." Although we do
not have all the details, we have heard of many success stories
about people using Cat's Claw.

In closing, I would like to share one person's experience with
Cat's Claw. This person said that for approximately the last 20
years he had been plagued by a chronic urinary tract problem
involving an unspecified inflammatory condition of the urethra
and other symptoms commonly associated with an enlarged
prostate gland. Throughout these years he visited a number of
different doctors, both allopathic and holistic. He tried conventional medicines, numerous vitamin and mineral regimens,
herbal remedy combinations, and an array of other natural
products—with minimal results.

In September of 1993, he was given an opportunity to sample

several ounces of Cat's Claw. He began experimenting with the herb by brewing it as a tea and drinking three cups a day. About halfway into his third day of doing this, he began to notice the chronic urinary symptoms starting to diminish. About halfway into the second week, the symptoms virtually were eliminated.

Since that initial experiment, as he continues to use Cat's Claw daily, his resistance to colds, flu, and other types of infection remains high; he now is able to perform heavier and more physically taxing work without the tired, sore muscles he normally would have experienced in the past.

Because of the numerous beneficial elements in this plant, the many years of use as a traditional medicine, coupled with his experience using this herb, he has come to believe that Cat's Claw has tremendous potential as a successful preventative, as well as a treatment for many of today's serious health problems.

According to available research, adults should take four capsules daily and children (under 12) should take three capsules daily as a preventative measure. Therapeutic amounts would be three to six grams daily. However, in some instances 20 grams might be used.

Since there has been such extensive research on this amazing plant, we feel Cat's Claw *(Uncaria tomentosa)* has great potential as a prevention for the serious health problems we face today.

We at Nature's Nutrition, Inc. are proud to bring you such a wonderful herb. You can obtain Cat's Claw for your good health by calling our office: 1-800-242-1115.

The choice is not difficult...but the choice is yours.

If you want to help alleviate premature aging and disease, take organic supplements and antioxidants such as The Capsule, Haridra, Cat's Claw, and O.E.F.

Additional organic nutritional supplements offered by Nature's Nutrition are:

• Total Veggies Plus—Organically grown green barley, broccoli, brussels sprouts, cabbage, carrots, cauliflower, garlic, and onions in easy-to-take capsules for those too lazy to eat their vegetables.

• Colon Cleanser/Detoxifier—Almost everyone who eats the Basic American Diet (BAD) has a colon impacted from improper eating habits.

• Awesome Energy—For those individuals who have that tired, worn-out feeling most of the time.

- Indian Olibanum—No need to suffer from arthritis pain.
- Slim-It—For those who need to lose weight.
- Anti-Radicals with Pycnogenol—Vitamins A, C, E, Selenium, SOD, and Pycnogenol, the most potent antioxidant formula.
- Pycnogenol-30 mg—The miracle antioxidant from the grape pips.
- Cold/Flu Formula—Chase those sniffles away.
- Germanium—Essential to human health.
- Green Barley Powder or Tablets—The most nutritious plant on earth.
- Coenzyme Q_{10}—For your heart's sake.
- Ginko Biloba—Cerebral vascular insufficiency, peripheral arterial insufficiency, and peripheral vascular diseases.
- PAK (Pyridoxine Alpha-Ketoglutarate)—Enhance physical performance.
- Milk Thistle—Detoxify and enhance liver function.
- Marine Lipid Oil (Fish Oil)—Reduce cholesterol and triglycerides. Reduces inflammation of arthritis.
- Lactobacillus sporogenes—Increases the natural microflora of the human gut. Aids in digestion, bowel regulation, and immunity.
- Montana Gold Flax Oil—Richest source of valuable Omega-3 fatty acid.

To obtain these marvelous organic food supplements, call our toll-free number: 1-800-242-1115.

Be happy—don't worry. Good health to you!

A Guide to Herbal Health Care/ The Beginning of Herbs

All herbs are a blessing from God. Nature's Nutrition herbs are pure, natural, and organic for *your* benefit.

Man has used herbs to treat sickness and disease for thousands of years. Herbs have been with us since the beginning of time. A majority of people in the world use herbs today, as they know of the benefits for their bodies. Herbs are very safe and reliable with no side effects. The Bible talks about the use of herbs for our health. In Genesis 1:29, God tells us, "Here I have given to you all vegetation bearing seed which is on the surface of the whole earth and every tree on which there is the fruit of a tree bearing seed. To you let it serve as food."

Nutritionists and herbalists of today help people build good health. THE PUBLISHER makes no medical claims for any-thing mentioned in this book, and it is not the intention to diagnose or prescribe. The information is offered for use in main-taining and promoting health, in cooperation with a physician. If you use the information in this material without a physician's approval, the person is diagnosing for himself. No responsibility is assumed by the authors, publishers, or distributors of this publication for use of the information contained herein in lieu of a doctor's services. No guarantees of any kind are made as to the performance or effectiveness of the preparations in this book.

Herbal Food Combinations for Your Good Health

Specific herbal formulas are listed for most conditions. These herbs have been found by ancient and modern practice to possess specific health restorative properties for the conditions mentioned. In compiling this information, we have used dozens of reliable herbal books from around the world.

Herbs are known to be a natural God-given food for the health of our bodies. The herbalist and nutritionist understands that only the body has the ability to heal itself. Herbs are an aid in the process of normalizing, rebuilding, and maintaining the proper function of the body. Herbs help the body stay healthy.

Acne—This formula helps to cleanse the blood. Beneficial for those suffering from acne, blackheads, pimples, etc.

Algazim—A bromalade rich in potassium, makes Vitamin A available to the body. Has been beneficial for cataracts.

Allergies—When the body's chemistry is balanced and receives the proper nutrients, many allergies improve.

Anemia—These herbs work with the kidneys to increase the flow of urine, restores the nutrients' salts, blood purifier, cleanses impurities from the blood.

Arthritis/Rheumatism—This combination of herbs helps to remove waste matter from the body, one of the leading causes of arthritis. Specifically designed to alleviate pain and stiffness associated with arthritis.

Asthma—When the body is cleansed of mucus and phlegm, asthma sufferers find great relief. Refrain from consuming mucus-forming foods, such as milk, sugars, cheeses, etc.

Backache—These herbs relax the muscles, ease the pain, and soothe the nerves, giving relief of back pain.

Blood Purifier—Your organs function better, you have more energy and vitality, and your skin will look better when the body's blood is pure, as God intended.

Bronchitis—These herbs cleanse the throat, ease the coughing attacks, and allow for free breathing. They also cleanse the stomach and bronchial tubes of mucus and phlegm.

Cholesterol—This herbal combination helps to prevent the deposit of dietary cholesterol on arterial walls, reverses the cholesterol build-up, reduces the risk of developing heart problems, and lowers the body's high serum cholesterol.

Circulation—Poor circulation inhibits the proper functioning of organs. These herbs allow an even flow of blood to all parts of the body, which is essential for good health.

Colds—This herbal formula will help break up the toughest colds in 24 hours.

Constipation—Constipation is not natural. It is essential that the bowels move several times daily for the entire system to work properly. These herbs eliminate waste from the body and keep the bowels regular for good health.

Coughs—This herbal formula is excellent for severe cases of coughing, bronchial or asthmatic. Puts the body in tune with good nutrition, cleansing and purifying the system.

Diabetes—These herbs are highly valuable in activating and stimulating the pancreas to its normal function, regulating the correct use of sugar in the bloodstream. Cleans out mucus and sediments and arrests infection in the pancreas.

Diarrhea—This herbal formula is more effective when taken with plenty of water. Exercise also is beneficial, such as walking.

Digestion—These herbs work magnificently with the body's natural digestive process. Relieves the distress associated with poor digestion, which is one of the most common causes of body ailment.

Ears—This herbal formula clears mucus and alleviates pain from ears, helps the eardrum, reduces swelling, helps relieve ringing, and loosens wax build-up.

Eye Strengthener—These herbs contain nutrients which bring relief to many eye problems, i.e. poor eyesight and cataracts. Beneficial when eyes are bloodshot, sore, swollen, etc.

Female Regulator—This herbal formula blends together the proper nutrients for the strengthening of all female organs. Beneficial in all female health problems.

Gall Bladder—This herbal formula is devised to fight the ill effects of gall stones and gall bladder trouble, strengthening the gall bladder.

Gout—Through this herbal formula, the proper nutrients are being put into the system, bringing relief from the pain associated with this arthritis-like affliction.

Hair—This herbal combination puts nutrients back into the hair and stimulates growth. Combats effects of contaminants on the hair.

Headaches/Migraine Headaches—Herbs that cleanse and strengthen the body, which are very helpful in acute and chronic headaches.

Heart—Herbs for the benefit of the heart, which strengthen and stimulate the heart, quiet and soothe the nerves, cleanse and tone body organs allowing less stress on the heart.

Heartburn—This herbal formula tones digestive organs, combats fermentation and gas, and invigorates the body's entire system.

Hemorrhoids—This herbal formula, which aligns the body's system with the proper nutrients, will alleviate hemorrhoid problems almost immediately.

High Blood Pressure—This herbal formula strengthens the blood vessels and quiets the body, steadily lowering the blood pressure.

Impotence—This herbal formula increases the sexual desire and the ability to perform sexually, while correcting conditions of impotence and strengthening sexual power.

Insomnia—This herbal formula will soothe the nervous system, ease tension, and induce relaxation and sleep in a natural way.

Intestinal—This herbal formula strengthens and lubricates the intestines, improves mucous membranes, soothing and healing gastrointestinal tract disorders.

Itching—This herbal formula is very beneficial for excessive itching.

Kidneys—This herbal formula will strengthen weakened kidneys. Lower back pain, failing to urinate, a general feeling of sluggishness and weakness can be an indication of weakened kidneys.

Liquor Habit—Desire to quit altogether is a must. This herbal formula will aid in the neutralization for the taste of liquor.

Liver—The liver is the filtering and detoxification organ of the body. This herbal formula will strengthen the liver and eliminate poisonous matter from the blood. Synthetic drugs and foods consumed do not allow the liver to work properly.

Lungs—This herbal formula performs beautifully for the unhealthy lungs.

Menopause—This herbal formula relieves the symptoms of menopause, i.e., irritation and frustration, nervous headaches, and hot flashes. Has a relaxing, soothing, and calming effect.

Menstruation Problems—This herbal formula is a must for women having difficulty with menstruation. Relieves cramps and regulates menstrual cycle and flow, alleviates nervous irritation, helps with congestion of female organs, and stimulates circulation.

Mental Alertness—This herbal formula provides essential nutrients to the brain. Increases and improves concentration, circulation, mental stamina, memory. Helps clarity of mind and promotes restfulness.

Minerals—A good overall tonic—aids in such ailments as hair loss, nail breaking, cramps in the legs, broken and weak bones, mental fatigue, kidney disorder, and rheumatism. Especially rich in natural calcium, B-12, silica, and trace minerals.

Motion Sickness—This herbal formula helps to combat nausea that results from motion. Relaxes the entire body, decreases anxiety. Absolutely no side effects.

Muscle Relaxant—Strengthens nerves and soothes muscle spasms, relieves muscle tension, increases blood flow to muscles for a beneficial effect on muscle pain.

Nerves/Revitalize—A fast-acting herbal formula for the worried or up-tight individual. Contains nutrients to feed and repair frayed nerve endings. This formula will rebuild and re-vitalize the entire nervous system when taken over a long period of time.

Pancreas—Nutrients in this herbal formula help to heal mucous membranes anywhere in the body, stimulates, regulates, and increases the activity of the pancreas. Contains herbs for kidney disease prevention.

Prostate Problems—This herbal formula helps relieve pain, inflammation, and infection of the prostate. Cleanses the prostate glands and stimulates urine flow when an enlarged prostate is inhibiting the flow.

Semen/Testes—This herbal formula gives renewed energy and new life to the male genitals. Energizes sexual glands, improves testosterone and rejuvenates the flow of hormones. Improves the genitals and nervous system. Increases sperm production.

Sinus/Hayfever—This herbal formula helps to break down and expel mucus, thus reducing congestion in and around both maxillary and frontal sinuses. Also, clears nasal passages and reduces eyeache from sinus trouble.

Skin—For a more vibrant and healthy looking skin, this herbal formula cleanses skin, helps improve dryness, improves skin tone, and relieves inflammation and irritation of the skin.

Smoking—This herbal formula helps to deter the taste for cigarettes, cleanses the blood, calms and relaxes nerves, and uplifts spirits. Tobacco smoke eventually ends up in the blood stream, which affects every tissue and organ of the body.

Varicose Veins—This herbal formula is very effective in strengthening the blood vessels and veins. It is imperative to purify and cleanse the blood to successfully recover from the difficulties of varicose veins. These herbs provide the necessary nutrients to cleanse the blood.

Water Retention—This herbal formula will eliminate poisons from the body by activating the kidneys, thereby reducing water retention. Reduces mucus accumulation in the body.

Individual herbs and herbal extracts are available upon request. All herbal food formulas are packaged 120 capsules to a bottle.

Dr. Tom Corbitt and Dr. Dee Corbitt

Drs. Tom and Dee Corbitt are Naturopaths, Master Herbalists, and Certified Clinical Nutritionists, Licensed by the State of Florida Department of Medicine.

— RESPONSE PAGE —

Save money and shop from the convenience of your home or office! No extra charge to use your MasterCard, VISA, or DISCOVER card. FREE shipping on all orders of 12 items or more within the 48 continental United States.

Telephone Orders: Call our toll-free number: 1-800-242-1115 and charge your order to your VISA, MasterCard, or DISCOVER card. Please have your account number and expiration date on hand.

☐ I read about Nature's Nutrition in Lindsey Williams' new book, *You Can LIVE!* Please send me a catalog with information about your products.

PLEASE PRINT:

Name _____

Street/Box No. _____

City/State/Zip _____

Phone (_____) _____

Mail inquiry to:

Nature's Nutrition
866 20th Place • Vero Beach, FL 32960
Fax: (407) 569-6501
Toll-Free Order Number 1-800-242-1115

Chapter 5

Nutrition the Biblical Way

By Mindi Carmack, Ph.D.

After the flood, the earth was a devastated wasteland. How would Noah and his family survive?

Biblical scholars agree that since the earth was desolate and nothing could grow, it was necessary to make a change in the dietary guidelines. Some of them maintain it was only a temporary injunction, valid until the fields would blossom forth again, but others say this was a permanent change. From this time on, they believe, it has been permissible to eat meat. This issue remains controversial, but we know that meat-eating began shortly after the Great Flood and became an established practice.

Today, we face a very serious problem since most of the meat is not fit for human consumption. The animals are fed growth hormones, steroids, and antibiotics, which remain in the meat when the animals are butchered, then enter the body when the meat is consumed.

In fact, more drugs are used by cattlemen than by medical doctors. The meat production enterprise requires over 2,700 drugs, including antibiotics, hormones, tranquilizers, and pesticides which are consumed in our meats today.

The USDA reported recently that "nearly four out of every ten chickens sold to consumers are contaminated by salmonella."

Millions suffer yearly from these contaminated meats; for

example, between 1971 and 1983, there were over 15 million estimated associations of salmonella illness with meat and poultry. Scientists estimate that about 30% of the 69 million to 275 million cases of diarrhea that occur each year result from food contamination.

Pork is highly contaminated. Pigs are to the animal world what the turkey buzzard is to the bird world. Pigs are scavengers by nature, which means they act like living garbage cans. They do the job they were created to do. No rotten carcass or rancid garbage remains where pigs root.

The Bible states in Leviticus 11:7: "And the swine, though he divide the hoof, and be clovenfooted, yet he cheweth not the cud; he is unclean to you."

Pigs cannot be divorced from their scavenger nature. As the Bible states, they are unclean for us. Pigs actually will eat their own feces, even in the most carefully controlled situations.

The danger of pork, improperly cooked, has been understood as trichinosis, caused by a parasite that can enter the body through pork that has been eaten. The pig's insides often are infested with trichinosis.

Trichinosis is transmitted first to pigs when they are fed uncooked garbage or when infested rodents, such as mice or rats, invade the pigs' feeding areas. A person becomes a host when, upon eating insufficiently cooked pork, the encysted larvae hatch in the intestines and migrate to encyst in muscles. Trichinosis is characterized by a flu-like illness, with severe muscle aches and pains, mimicking at least 50 other illnesses.

Smoked hams and sausage also can carry pork tapeworm infection if the pork tapeworm eggs migrate to the brain, where they will hatch into larvae and create cysticercosis, a condition that produces dementia, epilepsy, and sometimes death.

Overall, the pig is a very sick animal. Pigs do not grow old, due to the fact that their biological age is limited to a few years. They cannot live much beyond six years as breeders, since signs of cancer are unavoidable.

Now we understand why the Bible advises us not to eat pork.

Shellfish is another food that always have been scavengers by nature. Leviticus 11:9-12 tells us that these are the guidelines received by Moses concerning seafood. "These shall ye eat of all that are in the waters: whatsoever hath fins and scales in the waters, in the seas, and in the rivers, them shall ye eat. And all that have not fins and scales in the seas, and in the rivers, of all that move in the waters, and of any living thing which is in the waters, they shall be an abomination unto you: They shall be even an abomination unto you; ye shall not eat of their flesh, but ye shall have their carcases in abomination. Whatsoever hath no fins nor scales in the waters, that shall be an abomination unto you."

The smooth-skinned catfish is a scavenger. The best bait to catch him is rotten meat. If it is rotten and smelly enough, the catfish will eat it.

Crab, shrimp, lobster, oyster, and clams are also scavengers. Carcasses floating in the river are covered with crabs. Alongside the river you find people catching these same crabs and taking them home to feed their families.

Parasites are a common problem with scavengers. Oriental lung flukes come from raw or inadequately cooked fish, such as crabs and crayfish.

Most people have better sense than to eat scavengers. Dogs, cats, rats, skunks, turkey buzzards, wolves, bears, foxes, hawks, swine, sharks, and shellfish are best left alone. Their flesh contains a substance different from other animals, a strong chemical substance to cope with the carrion they eat. It makes their meat taste different.

The Bible requires us to stay healthy. It orders us to refrain from eating scavengers which may be diseased. "Health" in exchange for obedience!

As with meats and fish, dairy products now contain antibiotics, hormones, pesticides, radioactive isotopes, and other toxic materials, as well as—on occasion—disease-producing bacteria.

So, what causes dairy products to be unfit and unsafe to drink? Almost all milk is pasteurized. Pasteurization destroys about 38% of the Vitamin B-complex, lowers Vitamin B-12 by 12%, destroys Vitamins A and C, reduces the availability of calcium by 10%, lowers protein digestibility by 4%, protein biological value by 17%, and destroys the digestive enzyme phosphatase.

The pasteurization of milk also causes loss of iodine and lecithin, which is destroyed through splitting up of phosphoric acid, the casein (changes its reaction to acid and rennet), the lactose becomes caramelized, the citric acid is destroyed, the soluble calcium salts are transferred to an insoluble state, the carbonic acid is destroyed, and enzymes and vitamins also are destroyed.

When some of the minerals in milk, notably calcium and phosphorus, and some of the proteins of milk are altered physio-chemically by the pasteurizing process, the food value of the milk is reduced greatly.

Pasteurized milk was tested against raw milk at the Auchin Cruise Agricultural College in Great Britain, by feeding each to comparable groups of calves. Eight calves were fed pasteurized milk and eight were fed raw milk. Thirty days later at the completion of the test, six of the eight calves that were fed pasteurized milk had died, and the remaining two were unable to reproduce any offspring. Those fed raw milk all lived!

With this kind of testing being done, I would ask, "What is the real reason milk is pasteurized?" The purpose of pasteurizing milk is to hide the filthy sources. There are almost no sanitary requirements made upon the producers of pasteurized milk, for it is assumed that pasteurization will render all milk safe, even dirty milk; pasteurization prevents even dirty milk from souring, so that after many days of travel and storage, it still may be sold as "fresh." It also gives the milk a longer shelf life. The require-ment that all milk be pasteurized before being sold also provides a means of eliminating the small producer as a competitor of the larger dairy interests. It creates a milk monopoly. These are the real reasons that milk is pasteurized.

Another problem that makes milk unsafe and unfit to drink is the process of homogenization. Homogenized milk is one of the major causes of heart disease in the United States, reports Dr. Kurt A. Oster, M.D. Dr. Oster explains how homogenized milk triggers heart and circulatory disease in the following manner:

1. The milk homogenization process causes an enzyme called xanthine oxidase (XO) to become trapped within liposomes (very small, fat-like membranous globules).

2. After milk is consumed, stomach acid and gastric enyzmes digest and inactivate only some XO. Liposomes protect much of the XO from digestion. However, when non-homogenized milk is consumed, all XO is broken down during digestion.

3. Membrane bound packets of XO are transported through the intestinal wall into the circulatory system. White blood cells transport XO through the circulation.

4. XO attacks plasmalogen, a vital structural component of the cell membranes of cells in heart and artery wall tissue. Superoxide ($O-_2$) is produced during the reaction.

5. Superoxide initiates a chemical chain reaction which can produce lesions in artery walls or damage to the heart muscle itself.

6. Arterial lesions harden eventually into calcified plaques due to the disposition of minerals.

7. Cholesterol and fatty streaks cover calcified plaque and obstruct blood flow.

8. Circulation to remote areas of the body, such as the prostate gland, the eyes, the brain, and the skin is first affected.

9. Artery walls may lose their elasticity due to a large number of calcified plaques.

10. High blood pressure is one symptom of the loss in arterial elasticity. Angina (chest pain) results from a diminished blood flow through branches of the coronary artery. The combination of adrenaline (released during stress), caffeine, and nicotine may constrict a diseased coronary artery, depriving the heart of oxygen, triggering a heart attack.

The circumstantial evidence of homogenized milk can be summarized as follows:

1. The heart disease rate skyrocketed after the homogenization of milk became commonplace in the United States.

2. Xanthine oxidase destroys plasmalogen. In the arteries of heart disease victims, extensive plasmalogen tissue destruction is evidenced.

3. Active xanthine oxidase has been isolated from the plaques and lesions lining artery walls.

4. It has been demonstrated that biologically active xanthine oxidase can pass through the intestinal wall into the circulation within protective packets called liposomes.

5. Cow's milk xanthine oxidase has been identified in the human circulation through the presence of human antibodies to cow's milk xanthine oxidase.

6. Folic acid therapy has helped heart disease patients, since it blocks the action of xanthine oxidase and helps to rebuild

plasmalogen.

7. Female sex hormones inhibit xanthine oxidase. Therefore, arteriosclerosis is rare in women prior to menopause.

8. Male sex hormones chemically enhance xanthine oxidase activity. Arteriosclerosis and heart attacks are more common in men.

9. The heart disease death rate is, to a large part, proportional to the volume of homogenized milk consumed in each country. Circulatory disease is rare in countries in which whole (raw) milk is consumed.

10. Heat inactivates xanthine oxidase. Countries in which milk commonly is preboiled have relatively little heart disease.

Let's find out biblically what our options are to pasteurized cow's milk: Proverbs 27:27 states: "And thou shalt have goats' milk enough for thy food, for the food of thy household, and for the maintenance for thy maidens."

The Bible is very clear that we are to drink goat's milk. Goat's milk is a wonderful choice because it is closer in composition to human milk than cow's milk, in fact, I always recommend feeding infants goat's milk when the mother is unable to breast feed, because it is closer to human milk than any other milk, including man-made formulas.

Another alternative to pasteurized milk is raw cow's milk. The Bible states in Exodus 3:8: "And I am come down to deliver them out of the hand of the Egyptians, and to bring them up out of that land unto a good land and a large, unto a land flowing with milk and honey; unto the place of the Canaanites, and the Hittities, and the Amorites, and the Perizzites, and the Hivites, and the Jebusites." Isaiah 7:22 says: "And it shall come to pass, for the abundance of milk that they shall give, he shall eat butter: for butter and honey shall every one eat that is left in the land."

Raw milk nourished the spirits as well as the bodies of the biblical peoples. Milk and honey together symbolized good health, prosperity, and blessings from God. Milk and milk products were an important part of the daily diet in biblical times. However, it was difficult—if not impossible—to keep raw milk fresh in those days. The solution was to use the same fermentation process with milk as was used to make wine or sourdough bread. The result was what we know today as yogurt, cheese (soft and hard), and what is sometimes called curds in the Bible, but may have been butter—another milk byproduct. Butter seldom was used for cooking then. Olive oil was used, instead.

Raw milk has been called "the perfect food" because it provides so many of the nutrients we all need to grow, to fight off disease, and to stay healthy. For example, one cup of this "perfect food" contains:

Calories	157
Fat	8 gr.
Carbohydrates	11.9 mg.
Calcium	250 mg.
Protein	8.4 gr.
Potassium	406 mg.
Vitamin A	15% MDR*
Vitamin D	25% MDR*
Sodium	126 mg.

*Minimum Daily Requirement

All of these make raw milk an incredibly powerful and versatile health elixir, something that people of biblical times seemed to know instinctively, as stated in II Samuel 17:28,29: "Brought beds, and basins, and earthen vessels, and wheat, and barley, and flour, and parched corn, and beans, and lentiles, and parched pulse. And honey, and butter, and sheep, and cheese of kine, for David, and for the people that were with him, to eat: for they said, The people is hungry, and weary, and thirsty, in the wilderness."

It is no wonder that this "perfect food"—milk—was so important in the lives of biblical people who had to depend on natural foods as healing medicines.

The problems with consuming dairy products today have to do with what modern food technology has done to them.

What has modern technology done to our food supply? The last 50 years has seen—and there continues to be—toxic technology in agriculture.

Not many farm publications concern themselves with this issue. Almost all defend toxic technology the way the Medellin Cartel defends the international distribution of drugs.

Some farmers simply "turn off" when someone suggests that there is something wrong with chemical or organic synthesis in, on, and around the food supply.

According to USDA data, more than 80% of samples taken of peaches, apples, and celery contained residues of one or more pesticides. On just 12 fruits and vegetables tested, researchers found 13 carcinogens, 17 neutrotoxins, and 11 pesticides that disrupt the endocrine or reproductive system.

Three-quarters of a billion pounds of pesticides are sprayed on our foods annually! Eighty to one hundred million pounds of insecticides are eaten in the United States each year, and an average American consumes approximately 40 mg. of pesticides per year in food alone, and carries around about 100 mg. permanently stored in body fat.

It is estimated that every day 50,000 two-year-olds across America receive doses of pesticides that exceed the EPA's acceptable limits, and 1,500 of those children receive doses that exceed federal intake standards by a factor of ten.

Sixty to sixty-five percent of the residues are a threat to human safety. Some are approved by the FDA; some are foreign-made and, therefore, difficult to detect; and some are residues from formerly used pesticides, such as DDT.

Blood samples reveal that residual DDT (DDT was banned in 1972) still is contributing to breast cancer and reproductive defects in women. Now we have pesticides ten times as strong as DDT. Is there any question why the rate of diseases continues to escalate?

We need the vitamins and minerals fresh produce has to offer us, so what is the alternative to pesticide-laden produce? Organic farming!

Organic farming techniques recycle waste products and work in harmony with nature. Organic food may cost a little more because more of the work is done by hand, such as weeding. Also, the industry is still small, and organic farming is not subsidized to the same extent as conventional agriculture.

So, while pesticide-free foods cost more, the agony of illness and the high cost of medical treatment (which still may not cure the disease) is too great a price to pay. Just remember, good nutritious pesticide-free food can help you stay well.

If we go back to the times of the Bible, there were no such

things as pesticides, yet people seemed to live longer and healthier...probably because they left nature alone!

The Bible has a lot to say when it comes to the subject of sweeteners. In Proverbs 24:13 it states: "Eat honey, my son, for it is good; honey from the comb is sweet to your taste." Proverbs 25:16 says: "If you find honey, eat just enough—too much of it, and you will vomit." And Proverbs 25:27 declares: "It is not good to eat too much honey."

Why do we seek out sweet foods? When man gathered foods from the wild in the biblical days, sweet plants usually were safe in contrast to the bitter, which often were poisonous. It was probably man's instinct for the sweet taste that led him to seek out sweet fruits containing nutrients such as Vitamin C and natural, quick-energy-producing sugars.

For many reasons, mostly because it tasted so good, honey was one of the most popular foods among the people of the Bible. It became a symbol for abundance and God's blessings, thus "a land of milk and honey."

The people of the Promised Land consumed honey by itself as a food (the honeycomb) and used it to flavor and sweeten everything from soup to nuts!

Today, man is comsuming many refined food products that retain the sweetness, but not the nutrients.

Food companies know that Americans love them and, therefore, spend $100 million yearly to advertise foods on television. Half of them are sugary foods.

Sugar first was cultivated in India in 325 B.C., but remained a scarce luxury for many centuries. It became a common food only in the last 100 years.

Today, the average sugar consumption yearly in America is 125 pounds or 600 calories per day, at least 24% of the total diet, consumed primarily through thousands of prepackaged foods.

So, what are the effects of consuming refined sugar in such large amounts? Let us find out.

Sugar has been implicated in the following effects on bodily health:

1. Increased blood cholesterol and triglyceride levels that contribute to heart disease.

2. Unstable blood sugar levels that contribute to hypoglycemia,

diabetes, and aggravates criminal behavior.

3. Depletion of B-Vitamins stored in the body, which contributes to depression, an intensified craving for alcohol in alcoholics, and excessive estrogen in women that contributes to breast cancer.

4. Displacement of more nutritious foods with empty calories, contributing to obesity and lowered resistance to most health problems and degenerative diseases.

5. Upset of the homeostasis (balance) mechanism, which causes a perpetual craving for sugar—sugar addiction.

6. Increased uric acid in the blood, leading to gout.

7. Reduction of phosphorus in the blood that prevents bone calcification, and leeching of calcium from the bones, which contributes to osteoporosis.

8. Altered pH (acid/base) balance in the mouth, which causes tooth decay.

9. Reduced effectiveness of white blood cells to kill bacteria, thus encouraging infections.

According to *Polio Prevention,* by Duon Miller, sugar is a destroyer of health and classified as a drug, not a food. Technically, white sugar is $C_{12}H_{22}O_{11}$. Natural sugar in fruit is in a balanced combination with other constituents that enable it to be assimilated without damage, but when it is separated into a white, crystalline carbon substance called sugar, it is converted into alcohol almost immediately after it is taken into the body. It dehydrates the cells and leeches the calcium from the nerves, muscles, bones, teeth, and all tissues that are supplied with calcium and other alkaline elements. A serious calcium deficiency is a forerunner to polio.

What would be a good alternative to sugar? How about going back to the Bible? The biblical record for honey sets aside the argument that honey is no better than refined sugar. God's word is especially clear about this particular food. "Eat honey, my son, for it is good. . . . " but not too much. I wonder if God had the twentieth century in mind. He created honey as a whole, natural food with a wealth of nutritional value.

Honey contains 39% fructose, and it is also an important anti-fatigue food. Since it is predigested, it builds up alkaline reserves in the blood and tissues and provides a maximum of energy with a minimum of shock to the digestive system. Sugar-laden foods overload the bloodstream in 15 minutes; honey is absorbed over a period of four hours.

Honey contains B-Vitamins, Vitamin C, and at least 12 minerals. Honey is easily and rapidly assimilated, it provides a natural, gentle laxative effect, and is easier on the kidneys to process than all other sugars.

When honey is combined with whole grain flour or cereal high in dietary fiber and B-Vitamins, the body can digest honey very well without depleting stored nutrients in the body.

Honey, we now know, can kill bacteria and disinfect wounds and sores. Countless travelers have found that honey works when nothing else does to end the distress of traveler's diarrhea. Generations of grandmas have ordered hot honey to soothe sore throats. Honey seems to calm frayed nerves and, when life gets too stressful, it helps us get a good night's sleep. Asthmatics everywhere swear by honey's ability to help them breathe easier, which may be because the pollen in honey desensitizes and counteracts allergies.

Honey kills dangerous bacteria on the inside as well as the outside of the body. In the intestinal tract, it attacks and wipes out bacteria, especially those that cause diarrhea. In South Africa, for example, researchers found that honey did a marvelous job of eliminating such deadly diseases with diarrhea-related symptoms as salmonella, shigella, E. coli, and cholera. The study involved two groups of children being treated for acute gastroenteritis. All suffered terribly from diarrhea, brought on by intestinal infection. One group was given fluids mixed with honey; a second group, fluids mixed with sugar. Children who received the honey treatment recovered 40% faster than those who didn't.

The recommended antidiarrheal mixture is this: Pour 8 oz. distilled water and ¼ tsp. baking soda in a glass. In another glass, mix 8 oz. orange juice, a pinch of sea salt, and ½ tsp. honey. Alternate drinking from each glass.

For sore throats, folk medicine calls for a gargle of honey mixed with lemon juice or vinegar. This coats and lubricates the irritated linings of the throat, which make swallowing easier.

In 1958, D. C. Jarvis included several uses for honey in his bestselling book, *Folk Medicine*. Besides recommending honey as a treatment for such complaints as coughs, cramps, burns, and a stuffy nose, Jarvis also suggested, "A tablespoon of honey at the evening meal..." as a way of beating insomnia. Honey can lull you to sleep because of the natural sugars it contains. Biochemists now know that as our bodies burn sugar, a chemical substance called serotonin is produced by our brains. Serotonin's purpose is to relax us, quiet down all that brain chatter, and gradually put us to sleep.

Caution: The Center for Disease Control says we should not give honey to children under one year old. The reason is that botulism bacterial spores stick to honey. In adults, the immune system is mature and strong enough to fight off such attacks, but a child that young is not ready to take on such a powerful foe.

As with other good foods, honey can be refined. Heating over 160 °F and straining removes valuable bee pollen and some of the nutrients. Supermarket honey and a lot of it in health food stores are refined. The best quality honey is unheated, unfiltered honey. Be careful if the label on the honey says "uncooked," it does not classify as "unheated" because it can be heated to 160 °F and still be labeled "uncooked."

Honey can be stored indefinitely. Since heating honey destroys some of its nutritional value, heat it as little as possible when cooking over direct heat, adding it toward the last of the cooking process. When honey is used in baking, it is protected somewhat by being combined with other ingredients. Remember, though, the biblical warning in Proverbs 25:27 states for us "not to eat too much honey!"

You can do this by reducing the number of desserts and sweets you have. When you use honey in recipes, you only need to use half as much as white sugar. The strong flavor of honey curbs the appetite, too.

I get a lot of questions on artificial sweeteners. All I can say is, "Can man develop any imitation food that equals the nutritional life-giving value of God's original whole foods?" Unfortunately, Americans have turned to noncaloric sweeteners in order to cut down on sugars and calories. The best known artificial sweetener bears the tradename "Nutrasweet" (aspartame). Nutrasweet is made from phenylalanine, aspartic acid, and methanol (or wood alcohol).

What exactly are these components? Phenylalanine, when uncontrolled by Valkine or Turosine amino acids, causes seizures and brain damage. Phenylalanine is considered harmful to the unborn, and it causes facilitate seizures in children and adults. Also, millions of people carry a gene which makes them highly susceptible to the effects of phenylalanine without being aware of it. It also causes menstrual dysfunction, blocks serotopin in the brain (needed for balance), and raises the metabolism of pregnant women to three times the normal, resulting in severe retardation of offspring.

Aspartic acid is a neurotoxin, similar to glutamate, which was removed from baby food in the 1970's. When by itself, it is neurotoxic and known to cause endocrine disorders, brain tumors and death of brain cells, and is especially hazardous to the developing central nervous system of young children.

Methanol, the final component of Nutrasweet, is also known as wood alcohol, which is a highly toxic chemical that can affect any part of the body, particularly the brain and eyes. A teaspoonful has been known to cause death. Nutrasweet releases one molecule of methanol for each molecule of aspartame ingested. It then oxidizes into poisonous form, aldehyde and formic acid, which are know to cause cancer, genetic mutations, and birth defects. The symptoms of methanol poisoning, which is cumulative, unfortunately do not show up immediately and are almost too numerous to mention, but visual problems, blindness, lethargy, severe headaches, memory lapses, back pains, confusion, numbness, leg cramps, and gastric problems top the list.

Aspartame breaks down in liquid and when heated, it cannot be used for cooking. A number of chemicals into which it breaks down are very toxic, such as formaldehyde (a carcinogenic toxin) and DKP (connected with brain tumors).

The Food and Drug Administration (FDA) has registered five deaths caused by Nutrasweet. Eighty percent of the FDA's overall complaints about food additives concern Nutrasweet.

This are a list of symptoms commonly associated with Nutrasweet: headaches, dizziness, blindness, seizures, altered vision, memory loss, hearing loss, ringing in ears, balance problems, heart palpitations, muscle spasms, breathing difficulty, sleep problems, hives, rashes, vomiting/nausea, numbness, diarrhea, fatigue/weakness, abdominal pain, loss of taste, slurred speech, and depression.

The consequences of this noncaloric sweetener have been

disastrous. Nutrasweet is about 200 times sweeter tasting than a comparable amount of white sugar. By introducing Nutrasweet into your body, you decrease the amount of energy in the spleen and pancreas, and the immune system is depressed.

These noncaloric sweeteners do nothing to induce permanent weight loss. As you already can guess, the ability of the spleen and pancreas to transform foods will be hampered by the excessive quantity of sweet taste. In other words, it is possible for the digestive capacities to decrease each time you ingest Nutrasweet. The final result could be weight gain!

So, why hasn't something been done to ban this dangerous product? All one needs to do is follow the money trail and probe a little, and the answer becomes very simple and obvious. There are thousands of companies using Nutrasweet in diet sodas, Kool-Aid, Jell-O, tea, cocoa, juices, frozen desserts, puddings, cakes, cereals, candies, vitamins, medicines, etc. That equates to many billions of dollars in profits worldwide.

Is there an alternative to Nutrasweet? There is an herb that God created for us to use as a natural sweetener, and it's a wonderful alternative to Nutrasweet. It is called *Stevia*. Stevia is a natural sweetener, 30 to 100 times sweeter than sugar. Small amounts go a long way, and there is no aftertaste, as with sugar substitutes.

Research in Japan found Stevia to be nontoxic and safe to use. They use it in soy sauce, chewing gum, and mouthwash. It is a nonfattening sweetener and can be used in cold or hot cereals and in herbal teas. Stevia is high in chromium (which helps to establish blood sugar). It has manganese, potassium, selenium, silicon, sodium, and Vitamin A. It also contains iron, niacin, phosphorus, riboflavin, thiamine, Vitamin C, and zinc.

Quite impressive, isn't it? This herb gives you life and nutrition instead of robbing you of nutrients.

The Bible has a lot to say on the subject of herbs. They are mentioned in the Bible over 35 times. Hebrews 6:7 states: "For the earth which drinketh in the rain that cometh oft upon it, and bringeth forth herbs meet for them by whom it is dressed, receiveth blessing from God:. . . ."

Like all people of their day, the early Hebrews of the Promised Land were very familiar with all of the plants growing around them, especially herbs, which were used as medicine as well as food. The phrase, "garden of herbs," is used several times, so we know that biblical people set aside plots specifically for herbs.

I Kings 21:2 states: "And Ahab spake unto Naboth, saying, 'Give me thy vineyard, that I may have it for a garden of herbs, because it is near unto my house: and I will give thee for it a better vineyard than it; or, if it seem good to thee, I will give thee the worth of it in money.' "

The people of the Bible cultivated a variety of herbs for their healing powers, as well as the zestiness they added to otherwise bland food. Herbs and spices were necessary ingredients of almost every recipe, but I'm only going to mention a specific few from the scriptures.

Beginning with the Passover in Egypt, hyssop was referred to often in the Old Testament in connection with purification rites. David, for example, prayed to be purified with hyssop: "Purge me with hyssop, and I shall be clean..." (Psalm 51:7a).

Some modern scholars say that the hyssop of the Hebrew scriptures may have been a type of marjoram. This plant, part of the mint family, is common in Palestine. One variety of hyssop that grew abundantly in Israel and Sinai in biblical days still is used extensively by many people there today to flavor cooking and in medicinal teas.

The Romans brought hyssop from the Middle East to Europe, where even today hyssop tea is a standard home remedy for relief of rheumatism and respiratory complaints.

The hairs on the stem of the plant often are used to prevent blood from coagulating, which may explain why the Jews in Egypt were told to use it at the time of the Passover. "And ye shall take a bunch of hyssop, and dip it in the blood that is in the basin, and strike the lintel and the two side posts with the blood that is in the basin; and none of you shall go out at the door of his house until the morning" (Exodus 12:22).

The medicinal use of hyssop is found elsewhere in the New Testament, as John 19:29,30 states: "Now there was set a vessel full of vinegar: and they filled a spunge with vinegar, and put it upon hyssop, and put it to his mouth. When Jesus therefore had received the vinegar, he said, 'It is finished': and he bowed his head, and gave up the ghost."

In modern experiments, hyssop has halted the growth of the herpes simplex virus, which causes cold sores and genital herpes.

To support its age-old reputation as a decongestant and a remedy for the symptoms of colds and flu, scientists have found that the herb contains several soothing camphor-like substances which help loosen phlegm, so it can be coughed up more easily.

Another healing plant of the Bible was the olive. It was certainly one of the most valuable and versatile plant of biblical times and is mentioned frequently. Many passages contain references to olives, olive trees, olive yards, and olive oils. II Kings 18:31,32 says, "...then eat ye every man of his own vine, and every one of his fig tree, and drink ye every one the waters of his cistern: Until I come and take you away to a land like your own land, a land of corn and wine, a land of bread and vineyards, a land of oil olive and of honey, that ye may live, and not die: and hearken not unto Hezekiah, when he persuadeth you, saying, 'The LORD will deliver us.' "

Probably the most famous reference to olive oil and its healing powers is in the parable of the Good Samaritan, in which the Samaritan cares for a beaten and robbed traveler, treating his wound with oil and wine.

Olive oil is a high-energy food and one of the most digestible of all fats. The ancients of biblical times found ways to incorporate it somehow in nearly every meal, both for cooking and for table use. Olive oil can be mixed with wine and used to soften and soothe bruises and wounds, as in the parable of the Good Samaritan.

The "anointing with oil," which clearly was part of sacred tradition among biblical people, almost certainly was done with olive oil. One ancient piece of folk wisdom—which probably is as old as many parts of the Bible—tells us that "olive oil makes all your aches and pains go away."

A study, largely underwritten by the American Heart Foundation, found that on the Mediterranean island of Crete the mortality rate due to cardiovascular illness was the lowest in the world. They compared the figure—and the diets—with those of Finland and the United States, which have the highest rates of deaths from heart attacks.

The difference was in the types of fat in the diets. In countries with the highest rate of cardiovascular diseases, diets were heavy in saturated fats, which increased cholesterol levels. Monounsaturated fatty acids do not have cholesterol and olive oil contains

56% to 83% of these acids, also called oleic acids.

The trouble-making saturated fatty acids are found in animal fats, such as butter and lard. Fats, as any nutritionist will tell you, come in three groups. These are *saturated fats* (found in meat, butter, margarine, cheese, and chocolate), which raise blood cholesterol levels, and *polyunsataurated* and *monounsatu-rated fats* (from vegetables), which lower cholesterol.

A recent study found that LDL (bad) cholesterol levels can be reduced by 7% by substituting olive oil for margarine. In fact, margarine is made by processes which take the nutritious seeds from nature, press out the oil, process the oil (removing essential nutrients and producing altered and toxic molecules in the process), then harden the oil into margarine by over-heating, which chemically changes molecules, producing many new substances not found in natural foods or nature. In simpler terms, margarine is one molecule away from plastic!

Margarine also contains aluminum and nickel contaminants. Aluminum is particularly worrisome, because its presence in our body is associated with mental deterioration (Alzheimer's disease), with brittle bones (osteoporosis), and even with cancer.

Margarine contains almost no essential nutrients. It is mineral-poor, vitamin-poor, amino acid-poor, and essential fatty acid-poor. It contains no fiber. It contains no enzymes. Hence, it is a source of "empty" calories that make us fat and sluggish.

If you want to replace your margarine with butter, it is free of most of the altered molecules one finds in margarine. Butter is a natural substance. It contains small molecules (short chain fatty acids) not found in margarine, which feed bacteria that keep our intestine and colon healthy.

Butter, however, does contain cholesterol. While this was one of the main arguments in favor of margarine in the past, here too, new studies tell a different story. Cholesterol plays an important role in human health. It is required for making Vitamin D and sex hormones. It keeps cell membranes working properly, protects our skin, and produces bile acids which help us digest fats properly. Because of its importance to our health, our body makes what it needs if we don't eat any cholesterol.

But here is the kicker. It has been shown that even high cholesterol levels are not a problem for our heart and arteries if our foods provide us with sufficient antioxidants to keep cholesterol from becoming oxidized. Only oxidized cholesterol is damaging. Vitamins C and E are the key antioxidants that keep cholesterol from being oxidized into damaging forms.

Butter does taste better. It is free of toxic molecules produced by processing. It is free of aluminum, nickel, and other artifacts of industry. Butter does have some drawbacks. It may contain antibiotics and pesticides from food given to the cattle. It may contain hormones if these have been used. Like most margarines, it contains only a few essential fatty acids, substances that are required for health. These must be provided by seeds such as flax and sunflower seeds, or their oils. An excess of butter can crown out the essential fatty acids from their vital functions.

As a result, butter, though far superior to margarine for the maintenance of human health, should be used in moderation, alongside seeds and oils rich in essential fatty acids.

The best oil to use, of course, as the Bible states, "olive oil." It is the richest in monounsaturated fats. Four or five tablespoons of olive oil daily dramatically improves the blood profiles of heart attack patients. Two-thirds of a tablespoon daily lowered blood pressure in men.

If you are trying to reduce the amount of fat in your diet to avoid the risk of heart attack, think of olive oil as an ideal replacement. Anything you can sauté in butter, you can sauté in olive oil. Not only will you be helping your heart, but also pleasing your taste buds.

The healthy aspects of olive oil are not limited to its positive effect in the battle against heart disease. The evidence is strong that it also retards cancer growth. For example, olive oil seems to strengthen cell membranes, which makes them more stable and better able to resist the invasion of the "free radicals" that roam around the body causing so much damage. Lately, free radicals have become major suspects as a leading cause of cancer.

Olive oil is rich in Vitamin E, one of the best antioxidants available. Experts believe that those antioxidants help human cells fight off cancer. In doing so, they fortify the cells, thus slowing down deterioration that accompanies the aging process, since the cells are healthier and live longer. Incredibly, there is plenty of evidence to indicate that a diet rich in olive oil contributes to longevity. Olive oil has been shown to reduce the normal wear and tear of aging on the tissues and organs of the body and the brain. There also may be more to the connection between olives and longevity, because olive trees themselves have been known to survive for 3,000 year, and perhaps longer!

Olive oil has been shown to reduce gastric acidity. It protects against ulcers and aids the passage of food through the intestines, thus helping to prevent constipation. It also stimulates bile secretion and provokes contraction of the gallbladder, reducing the risk of gallstones. Since olive oil contains Vitamin E and oleic acid, which also are found in human milk, it aids normal bone growth and is most suitable for both expectant and nursing mothers, because it encourages development of the infant's nervous system before and after birth.

Since olive oil works wonders at blocking the tendency of blood to clot, improving good HDL cholesterol levels and reducing the dangerous buildup of bad cholesterol in arteries, some experts now strongly recommend olive oil as an excellent way to cut the risk of heart attacks and strokes.

The best kind of olive oil to get is "extra virgin" olive oil. It may cost a little more, but it contains more of those natural ingredients credited with fighting heart disease. A scientist advises that the purer the oil, the more you will be helping your heart.

Deuteronomy 8:8 states: "A land of wheat, and barley, and vines, and fig trees, and pomegranates; a land of oil olive, and honey;. . . ." As you plainly can see, olive oil has been well-spoken of in the Bible, and many years of research has proven the Bible to be right about olive oil.

We have seen many lives of men, women, and children who have been blessed because they used God's plants and proper nutrition.

Many of our clients have tried all of the common treatments offered by conventional medicine—expensive and many time dangerous drugs, surgery, etc., and after all this, they still were not well.

Our approach is very gentle; we let the Holy Spirit guide us in teaching you what the Creator had in mind for you all along. We recommend a proper diet of organic foods, herbs, and supplements that stimulate your body's defense system, so that the body is allowed to heal itself.

We all were designed to be healthy in body, mind, and spirit—

immune to illness, free of today's ravages of aging, full of energy, alert and creative, naturally happy and free of stress. You can have all of this and more when you follow what God planned for you. I wish you health and happiness, and may God bless you immensely! "...and the fruit thereof shall be for meat, and the leaf thereof for *medicine*" (Ezekiel 47:12).

— RESPONSE PAGE —

Dear Dr. Carmack,

I read about "Nutrition the Biblical Way" in Lindsey Williams' new book, *You Can LIVE!*

Please send me more information on your...

    ☐ Computer analysis test

    ☐ Muscle response monitor test

    ☐ Product line of herbs and supplements

    ☐ Availability for lectures

Thank you!

PLEASE PRINT:

Name _____

Address _____

City/State/Zip _____

Telephone (_____) _____

Please make your selection(s) and send to:

THE GOOD HERB
P. O. Box 5051
Glendale, AZ 85312-5051
(602) 504-0837

Chapter 6

Swedish Flower Pollen
The "Bee-Free" Flower Pollen Story

By B. P. Poovaiah, Ph.D.

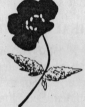

Dedicated to the Promotion of Nature's Most Perfect Food

From early history when the father of medicine, Hippocrates, said, "Let your food be your medicine and medicine be your food," pollen has been known to have a remarkably positive influence on the human body. Still, most people are unaware of the story behind pollen, and the new heights to which modern science and technology has taken it, for our ultimate good. Consider how life is sustained with pollen. Animals live off plants, and plant life begins with fertilization by these microscopic pollen grains. Pollen contains more important biofactors and nutriceuticals essential to life than any other nutrient source.

Support for pollen as a "perfect food" reference comes from the nutrients found to be present in the pollen itself. There are a number of basic elements in the human body—enzymes, hormones, vitamins, amino acids, and others, all of which must be renewed by nutrient intake. No one food contains them all—except pollen. Scientists have identified over 22 amino acids, all of the important minerals, and many enzymes in pollen. It also contains numerous vitamins, including A, C, D, E, and B-Complex.

The highly complex pollen molecule is the richest full-spectrum source of trace elements, fatty acids, nucleic acids (DNA, RNA), coenzymes, and prostaglandin precursors (a group of hormone-like compounds) found in nature. In total, pollen contains well over 100 biologically active compounds, and new elements continue to be discovered, with more new implications for the health of mankind. Some well-respected scientists believe that pollen contains *every* substance needed to maintain life. So, in that sense, pollen may, indeed, be the "perfect food."

HEALTH BENEFITS

Most of the health benefits claimed by proponents of pollen can be attributed to the fact that many of its elements act as catalysts. For example, natural vitamins, minerals, enzymes, and unidentified "life-giving" nutrient factors in pollen help the body to better digest, absorb, and assimilate the elements of food that otherwise would be eliminated as waste.

Researchers have reasoned, therefore, that pollen helps build up one's immune system. This, in turn, prevents many illnesses that result from low resistance, including allergies, colds, and viruses. Around the world, it's a pretty well-accepted axiom that "any food which builds health and prevents disease, may also heal disease in therapeutic levels." While biological medicines and common sense both teach us that this is true, in America, the Food and Drug Administration (FDA) forbids limits claims for any food, although no such prohibition exists in other countries.

It is interesting to note that a large percentage of the oldest people in remote parts of the world have been beekeepers, who kept for themselves the darkest (pollen-rich) honey at the bottom of the bee hives.

Pollen also has been found to help in weight reduction. Because it promotes digestion and absorption, pollen decreases the urge to eat. By feeding the glands with vital nutrients that normalize metabolism, loss of weight can occur.

Pollen's reputation for extra vim, vigor, and vitality is legendary. As the male sperm of the plant kingdom, pollen provides those biofactors that are precursors for sex hormones and micro-

Nature's Most Perfect Food

Chemical Analysis of Flower Pollen Extract:

Vitamins:
Provitamin A
  (carotenoids)
B 1 Thiamine
B2 Riboflavin
Niacin
B6 Pyridoxine
Pantothenic Acid
Biotin
B12
  (Cyanocobalamin)
Folic Acid
Choline
Inositol
Vitamin C
Vitamin D
Vitamin E
Vitamin K
Rutin

Carotenoids:
Beta-carotene
Xanthophylls
Zeaxanthin
Lycopene
Crocetin

Minerals:
Calcium
Phosphorus
Potassium
Sulphur
Sodium
Chlorine
Magnesium
Iron
Manganese
Copper
Iodine
Zinc
Silicon
Chromium
Molybdenum
Boron
Titanium

Enzymes:
Class: Oxidoreductases (24 in number)
Class: Transferases (21 in number) Class
Hydrolases (32 in number)
Class: Lyases (10 in number)
Class: Isomerases (5 in number)
Class: Ligases and Others (2 in number)

Fatty Acid Profile: Number of C-atoms and double bonds
Caprylic (C-6)
Capric (C-10)
Lauric (C-12)
Myristic (C-14)
Myristoleic (C-14) one double bond
Pentadecanoic (C-15)
Pentadecenoic (C-15) one double bond
Palmitic (C-16)
Palmitoleic (C-16) one double bond
Heptadecanoic (C-17)
Heptadecenoic (C017) one double bond
Stearic (C-IX)
Oleic (C-1#) one double bond
Linoleic (C-1#) one double bond Linolenic
(C-1#) two double bonds Arachidic (C-2())
Eicosenoic (C-20) one double bond
Eicosadienoic (C-20) two double bonds
Eicosatrienoic(C-20)three double bonds
Arachidonic (C-20) four double bonds

Long Chain Hydrocarbons:
n-pentacosane   Myo-inositol
n-heptacosane   Pinitol
n-nonacosane   Sequitol
n-tricosane

Growth Regulators:
Auxins
Brassins
Gibberellins
Kinins

Different Classes of Lipids in Flower Pollen:
Polar lipids
The major fractions of the polar
lipids in flower pollen are lecithin,
lysolecithin, phosphoinositol and
physphatidylcholine.

Neutral lipids
Monoglycerides
Diglycerides
Triglycerides
Free fatty acids
Sterols
Hydrocarbons

Dietary Essential Amino Acids and Physiological Essential Amino Acids:

Dietary Essential:	Physiologically Essential:
Histidine	Alanine
Isoleucine	Alpha-Amino-Butyric-Acid
Leucine	Arginine
Lysine	Asparagine
Methionine	Aspartic Acid
Phenylalanine	Cysteine
Threonine	Cystine
Tryptophan	Glutamic Acid
Valine	Glutamine
	Glycine
	Hydroxyproline
	Proline
	Serine
	Tyrosine

Low Molecular Weight Sugars and Related Compounds:

Fructose	Glucose
Mannose	Xylose
Galactose	Xylitol
Arabinose	Xylogalacturonan
Ribose	Glucoronolactone
Fucose	Raffinose
Hexasamine	Stachyose
Rhamnose	Sucrose
Maltotetralose	
Maltose	
Maltotriose	
Callose	

Others:

Chlorophyll	Nucleosides
Nucleic Acids	Vernine
Phenolic Acids	Guanine
P. hydroxybenzoic	Xanthine
P. coumaric	Hypoxanthine
Vanillie	Nuclein
Protocatechuic	Amines
Gallic	Hexodecanal
Ferulic	Pentosans
Terpenes	

Unknown:
Some of the greatest values of
Flower Pollen may stem from
elements which are for the moment
still unknown to science, and from
the synergistic action of all the
elements working together. IMPOR-
TANT: There are established
Recommended Daily Allowances for
many vitamins and minerals and
Flower Pollen contains trace
amounts of these ingredients. There
is no RDA or established need for
the majority of ingredients listed in
this Chemical Analysis

Prostaglandins:
A group of hormone-like compounds
derived from linoleic and arachidonic
acids that influence innumerable
body processes.

Phytosterols:
Fucosterol   Campesterol
Beta-sitosterol   Estrone
Stigmasterol

Flavonoids:
Quercetin   Apigenin
Kaempferol   Dihydroxquercertin
Isorhamnetin   Dihydrokaempferol
Narigenin   Myricetin
Luteolin

nutrients essential for healthy reproduction. Animal breeders in
Europe pay top dollar for pollen concentrates that are added
to stud food, dramatically increasing sperm count and sexual
activity in the animals.

It is important to understand that the term "perfect," as used herein to describe pollen, should not imply that bee pollen is without its problems. As beneficial as pollen is to so many people around the world, many who have tried it have experienced some allergic reaction. Users of bee pollen generally are not aware that it contains *some* degree of infestation. Additionally, many environmentalists find the price paid by the bee, i.e., lost legs and wings, to be distasteful and unacceptable.

HOW NATURE'S "PERFECT FOOD" BECAME EVEN MORE PERFECT

Over 50 years ago in Sweden, pollen researchers developed the theory that the secrets of life were in the pollen grains. They also observed that bees, among other reasons, collect pollen to create "royal jelly," the superfood that is fed only to the queen bee. They believed that it was this superfood that gave the queen bee the ability to grow to *three times* the size of other bees, and enjoy up to *thirty times* the lifespan of other bees who don't get the "royal" treatment. It was their opinion that this royal jelly made the difference between a worker bee and a queen bee—not genetics.

Swedish scientists invented the original bee pollen trap, similar to those still used by beekeepers today, but it soon was ascertained that the bee traps not only robbed the bees of an essential food, but also caused many bees to lose legs and wings on their way through the trap. Subsequently, pollen harvesters that *don't require bees* were invented, an innovative electromechanical technology that allows the harvesting of tons of "bee-free" pollen every year, directly from flowers.

There was still one more problem to overcome. These scientists believed that pollen had many health benefits, but they could not use the harvests of bee pollen to conduct medical studies to *prove* pollen's value, because they were unable to control the bees, as to what type of pollen they brought back from their travels. Without quality control, there could be no credible or reliable scientific research of the benefits. Also, they would be unable to achieve the standardized finished product they sought.

In addition, the secrets of the microscopic pollen grain had to be unlocked, because it was the *heart* of the pollen *inside* the indigestible husk that the bees sucked out through small openings that enabled them to make the royal jelly. A team of researchers eventually discovered that by dissolving the membrane over the openings, enzymatically, they were able to achieve the extraction of the pure pollen essence. They found that this raw pollen extract was too rich for human consumption, and the molecule was too complex for digestion. So, once again taking cues from the bees who mix their saliva with pollen extract to *predigest* it as royal jelly, the pollen scientists successfully developed a microbiological process for breaking down the raw pollen molecule into more assimilable water-soluble and fat-soluble components.

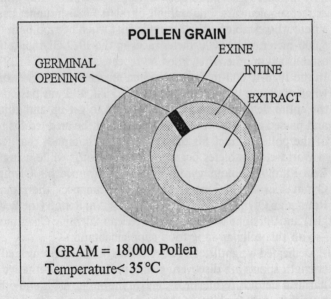

FIRST GENERATION FLOWER POLLEN EXTRACTS

Now that the pollen scientists had their quality controls in place, the scientific community worldwide began their testing in earnest.

Double blind studies were conducted with army troops in northern Sweden, demonstrating that the pollen extracts were effective not only in minimizing the symptoms of colds, flu, and upper respiratory tract infections, but also in *aiding quick recovery* after onset. It also was reported widely in Europe that the use of a flower pollen extract ointment met with unusual success when applied to skin rashes.

To this day, these pollen extracts are used extensively by European and Japanese physicians for correcting the nutritional deficiencies associated with certain prostate problems and other conditions of the reproductive organs. Clinics in a variety of countries around the world have used it for the full spectrum of health conditions. Perhaps the greatest reputation for pollen is for athletic performance. Many world-class athletes clearly have increased their endurance and strength when taking pollen extract supplements. One example of this is Finnish runner Lasse Viren, who established an Olympic first when he won both the 5,000-meter and 10,000-meter races in the 1972 Olympics. He established another first when he repeated these wins in 1976. In the 1976 10,000-meter race, Viren amazed the sports world when, well into the race, he tripped and fell, and was passed by the entire field of runners. He managed to get up and going, and passed everyone to win the race. Later, he credited his use of the pollen extract for the stamina to accomplish that feat.

World-class athletes began breaking records while using it. Bela Karolyi, famous gymnastics coach, trained his Olympic Gymnastics Champions—from Nadia Comaneci, the famous Romanian Olympic Champion, to Mary Lou Retton (the Revco girl) and Julianne McNamara, American Olympic Champions —with this cellular superfood supplementation.

Dedicated weightlifters, bodybuilders, and others engaged in strength sports are discovering that pollen is an alternative to harmful steroids. While providing all the amino acids and other nutrients that combine in the body to create superior steroid alternatives, it does so without harmful side effects.

Yet, perhaps saying it best is the research by Sir Alec Isaac, the English scientist who discovered interferon. Supposedly, during the last two years of his life, Dr. Isaac researched this pollen extract and discovered that it penetrated the membrane that protects the nucleus of the cell, combining with the DNA and RNA in the cell nucleus, helping in the process of synthesizing interferon for the body's immune system!

This is perhaps the biomedical breakthrough of the century because interferon is the body's first line of defense *(and offense) against disease. It is clearly one of the most important keys to the promotion* of good health and the *prevention* of disease. In fact, the volumes of research from around the world were so overwhelming regarding the health benefits of pollen extracts that the courts of Sweden actually cleared this product in a court case as a nutritional product in Sweden for which health claims could be made.

SECOND GENERATION FLOWER POLLEN EXTRACTS

Meanwhile, in Sweden pollen researchers continued their work and now have developed a dramatically improved "2nd generation" pollen extract, with distinct advantages over earlier extracts. These new extracts are more *pure,* more *potent,* and even more *perfect.*

Today, in quiet, remote countrysides in southern Sweden, selected varieties of flowers are grown for their best nutritional quality and balance. When the flower pollen reaches just the right balance of nutrients and maturity, the pollen grains are harvested by special electromechanical devices. These harvested pollen grains are purified and treated with special enzymes to break down the pollen sac and the long-chain molecules. An ultrasonic treatment is utilized to separate the pollen nutrients. These released nutrients are concentrated further and standardized under a cold processing technique to ensure that all of the vital nutrients (vitamins, minerals, amino acids, enzymes, RNA, DNA, building factors, carotenoids and other pigments, plant hormones, antioxidant factors, unsaturated fatty acids, prostaglandin precursors, and phytosterols) are preserved at proper balance. This concentrated, standardized pollen extract is sometimes referred to as "pollen essence."

The most recent scientific research with Swedish flower pollen extracts has focused on combining the concentrated, standardized, state-of-the-art 2nd generation pollen "essences" imported from Sweden, with other select nutrients, antioxidants, and special varieties of synergistic herbs, creating what some are referring to as a powerful "3rd generation" flower pollen formulation.

WHAT MAKES THESE 3rd GENERATION "POLLEN-PLUS" FORMULAS SO SPECIAL?

• *No bees are involved* in the collecting of the raw pollen.

THE EVOLUTION OF POLLEN – A SUMMARY

Pollen has come a long way as nature's most perfect food. It was half a century ago that Swedish scientists invented the original bee pollen trap. They soon learned the limitations of bee pollen—that it was contaminated, largely indigestible, lacking quality controls and thus impossible to work with on a scientific basis. So in the early 1950's they invented a pollen harvesting machine that didn't require the bees. For the next decade a team of researchers worked to develop the first generation pollen extract.

During the 70's and 80's, they continued their research, developing a second generation flower pollen extract with international patents on harvesting to control quality (without bees), extraction to improve assimilation (without the husk), and processing to remove allergens (without chemicals).

BEE POLLEN	1st GENERATION POLLEN EXTRACT	2nd GENERATION POLLEN EXTRACT
CONTAMINATED Bee pollen is graded by the level of contaminants found in bee pollen traps, including bacteria, mites, fungi, insect debris, rodent defecants, etc.	**SEMI-PURE** Although contaminants from bee pollen traps have been eliminated via mechanical harvesting, chemical residues from extraction processes remain.	**PURE** All chemical and bee contaminants have been eliminated via state-of-the-art harvesting, extraction and processing bio-technology.
NON-STANDARDIZED Bees cannot be controlled as to what pollens they carry back to the hive. Bee pollen will vary in quality from batch to batch and even tablet to tablet.	**SEMI-STANDARDIZED** Although pollen has been collected without the bees, the source of pollen harvested is not owned and quality controls vary with the source of supply.	**STANDARDIZED** The means of harvesting is owned and source of supply thereby controlled, insuring quality controls for consistent product standards.
UNCONCENTRATED Bee pollen is not a concentrated pure pollen product. It contains the hard outer husk which is virtually indigestible.	**SEMI-CONCENTRATED** Although the husk has been removed, extraction is not total; plus, the microbiological digestion (with chemicals) is not complete.	**CONCENTRATED** The husk is totally removed with a new pollen shredding process that makes for total extraction; plus the molecular predigestion (with enzymes) is complete.
ALLERGENIC More than 126 varieties of fungi and bacteria have been identified lodging in the coarse husks of bee pollen. A large percentage of people are allergic to bee pollen.	**SEMI-ALLERGENIC** Although the husks have been removed from the minute pollen grains, certain chemical residues and "undigested" molecules remain, RAST® tests are not performed, and allergies have been reported.	**HYPO-ALLERGENIC** Non-chemical processes for breaking down the complex pollen molecule into more assimilable components are employed. RAST® tests are utilized.
UNTESTED As an uncontrolled nonstandardized substance, scientific tests with any reliability are impossible with bee pollen.	**SEMI-TESTED** Although certain standards in harvesting and processing are met, the bio-technology processes used were engineered 18 years ago and do not meet current standards with new bio-technology.	**SCIENTIFICALLY PROVEN** The standardized pollen extract is produced under strict pharmaceutical regulations and newest technology. All ingredients fulfill the demands of scientific documentation. The factory (Swedish) follows GMP standards and is inspected by Swedish authorities annually.

- The pollen is mechanically harvested from *select varieties* of flowers, grown especially for their exceptional nutritional value.
- It is processed in *Sweden* by Swedish scientists.
- They contain *no infestations of any kind,* unlike "bee" pollen.
- It is *free* of pesticides, fungicides, and other pollutants.

- It is *more concentrated,* thus making it more potent.
- They contain special blends of select varieties of flower pollen essences, balanced with other select nutrients, making these formulas *truly unique* in the current market place.

The Swedish flower pollen extracts used are protected under international patents for *harvesting* without bees (for quality control), *extraction* without chemicals (to improve assimilation), and *processing* with live enzymes.

ENERGY FORMED—VITALITY RELEASED

Flower pollen has gained a world-wide reputation as an energy and vitality food for honeybees. Anyone who has watched them perform and observed their energy levels at least can begin to appreciate the pollen's energy-giving potential. No doubt, with this high-energy level of bees in mind, 3rd generation, high-energy flower pollen products are being developed, some with powerful antioxidants, other select nutrients, and a full spectrum of synergistic herbs. This makes it possible to achieve the very best from both the pollen and the herbs, as well as the other nutrients. These unique formulas energize your body chemistry to its maximum potential and work as "catalysts" in your body —meaning they work with existing body chemistry. In our bodies there are two basic energy-generating mechanisms, namely the metabolic pathways of *glycolysis and the Krebs cycle.*

With the help of these energy-releasing "pathways," food is biochemically and enzymatically converted into *energy, carbon dioxide,* and *water.* These pathways consist of hundreds of enzymes and coenzymes which are very specific in their activity of converting different food components into energy. These enzymes and coenzymes need certain specific nutrients and activators in order to perform this function. Nutrients in the pollen assist in this enzymatic reaction, thus completing the energy-releasing cycle. The energy released from this "energy cycle" is stored in the body in the form of ATP's (adenosine triphosphates) and creatine phosphate (CP). These are energy *powerhouses!* Potentially, flower pollen nutrients help unlock the ATP mechanism and release energy which, in turn, makes *you* feel *energized.*

THE ENERGY MACHINE
GLYCOLYSIS

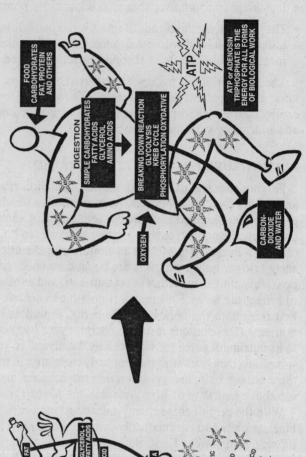

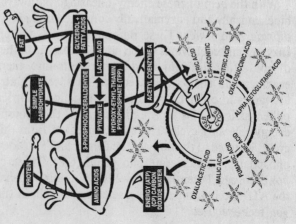

POLLEN-PISTIL DYNAMICS

Pollen grains contain energy stored in a pattern similar to atoms. Unlocking the energy from pollen is the key to success, and the best possible method is pollen fertilization with the pistil. Swedish scientists, after a quarter-century of research, introduced a method wherein hand-harvested female flower pistils were fertilized with the corresponding male pollen in special climate-controlled "incubators" to produce viable SOD (superoxide dismutase), a class of proteins having the common feature that they speed the dismutation of the superoxide radical. Researchers described this as "the greatest release of energy in the plant kingdom." The result is a biological transformation of pollen's rich blend of all vitamins, minerals, amino acids, enzymes, RNA, DNA, building factors—*virtually all of life's essential factors*—into an anti-aging, free radical scavenger system.

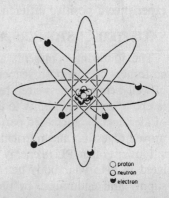

○ proton
○ neutron
● electron

WHAT TO EXPECT FROM POLLEN-RICH NUTRIENTS

- Helps give you *prolonged release* of natural energy.

- *Catalyst for enzyme "reactions"* that generate ATP (adenosine triphosphate) from energy cycle.

- Acts as a coenzyme and activator to help generate ATP, *the natural energy fuel*.

- Assists your immune system, *providing vital micronutrients*.

- Acts as an antioxidant *(prevents onset of free radicals)*

- Assists in *cellular rejuvenation* and rebuilding processes.

- Helps release your body's untapped energy to work for you— *less tiredness*.

- Improves quality *and* length of life.

Pollen nutrients work with your body, stimulating and helping to release your own natural forces, thereby allowing you to experience a positive difference in the way you feel.

SATISFIED CUSTOMERS ARE ENJOYING...

The following comments are what we hear from satisfied customers: "More positive mental outlook," "Increased feeling of well-being," "Less sleep required," "Higher overall energy levels," "Increased ability to accomplish tasks," "Higher level of alertness," "Increased performance in athletics," and "Improved digestion and nutrient assimilation."

Flower Pollen-PLUS energy formulas are scientifically formulated to help your body better utilize its own natural energy supply and endurance, by providing building blocks for the body's natural energy molecule, ATP. When needed, your body splits the ATP molecule, releasing molecular energy to work for you.

The purpose of this information is to assist you in making your own decisions about your health, not to suggest a substitute for any treatment that may have been recommended or prescribed by your physician. If you have medical problems, it is wise to seek out a medical professional knowledgeable in both traditional and alternative medical treatments.

B. P. Poovaiah, Ph.D.

Dr. Poovaiah is recognized widely as one of the leading authorities in America on Human Nutrition. His academic achievements include: B.S. degree in Agriculture and Animal Sciences, M.S. degree in Horticulture and Botany, M.S. degree in Food Technology and Food Science, Ph.D. in Human Nutrition from the University of California, Berkeley, and post-doctoral work in Dental Science at the University of California Medical Center, San Francisco.

Dr. Poovaiah also is respected widely within the scientific community and industry for his pioneering work in clinical studies. At the U.S. Department of Agriculture—Western Human Nutrition Research Center in San Francisco, his responsibilities included conducting biochemical research related to nutrient interaction, dietary fiber, and essential fatty acids. Working with large corporations, such as Cernitin America, General Foods, Shaklee, and Phillips Laboratory, Dr. Poovaiah's responsibilities included research, product development, and management.

— RESPONSE PAGE —

Dear Dr. Poovaiah:

I read about Swedish Flower Pollen Extracts in Lindsey Williams' new book, *You Can LIVE!*

Please send me more information on the "3rd Generation" Flower Pollen-PLUS developments about which you have written, and where I can purchase them.

Thank you.

PLEASE PRINT:

Name _____

Address _____

City/State/Zip _____

Telephone (_____) _____

Complete the form above and mail to:

Dr. B. P. Poovaiah
P. O. Box 237
Tallmadge, OH 44278

Chapter 7

The Mystery of Aloe Solved

By Robert M. Siegel, M.D., F.A.A.P.

For decades the medical community has all but discounted the idea that edible plants or plant molecules have any potential for supporting and enhancing the natural healing process. However, researchers now are discovering that certain plant substances, called phytochemicals, not only support healing, but actually trigger various functions of host defense.

THE CUTTING EDGE OF DISEASE-PREVENTION RESEARCH

A recent article in *Newsweek* stated, "Just a few years ago, scientists didn't even know phytochemicals existed. But today, they are the new frontier in cancer-prevention research."

My life was changed forever by what I consider to be the most significant of these discoveries, and I now am committed to tell that story to all who will listen. Eight years ago, the surgeon who had just completed exploratory surgery on my brother brought me the worst possible news I could have imagined. My brother's prostate cancer had spread throughout his body and the prognosis was terminal. I began dialoguing with the nation's leading cancer experts, only to discover that there were no good treatments available. As a last resort, I contacted a colleague of mine, Dr. Reg McDaniel, who had been contracted by a pharmaceutical company researching the active or functional component in the aloe vera plant. Dr. McDaniel encouraged my brother to begin taking this newly discovered and stabilized aloe product with his standard medical treatment. I honestly gave this no chance, but realized that my brother had no options left. I knew Dr. McDaniel, who had served as Chief of Pathology and Chief of Staff of a major metroplex hospital, was extremely confident in the potential of this treatment program.

To my utter amazement, my brother's condition began to improve immediately. Today, he is totally free of cancer and is, in fact, playing tennis better than ever before. Any doctor who has seen his CAT scans is shocked at the turnaround.

Eight years ago, this plant-origin therapeutics/prevention concept was totally foreign, but today, prestigious research facilities such as the National Cancer Institute and Johns Hopkins University are doing exciting research on the various phytochemicals found in certain fruits and vegetables. Unlike vitamins and minerals, these unique plant compounds are being classified as "functional components," which means they have the potential to prevent disease.

These newly discovered phytochemicals are on the cutting edge of cancer research. Each plant phytochemical appears to have a targeted effect on the body's defense system. The "functional component" in aloe vera, however, seems to be a master orchestrator of the immune response. Research has shown its capability to up-regulate and down-regulate the immune response and to enhance the activity of other bio-active substances.

The following is the story of the doctors who discovered and patented this amazing molecule. They endured years of ridicule to become the leading experts in this fast-emerging field of nutraceutical compounds.

ALOE'S SECRET MOLECULE DISCOVERED

In 1979, while working as a candidate for his doctoral degree in pharmacology at the University of Texas Health Science Center in Dallas, Bill McAnalley, Ph.D., started his scientific investigations of the aloe plant. His goal was to settle the medical controversy of whether the gel of the aloe plant, long esteemed in folk-medicine, actually had medicinal properties. The initiator and provider of funds for this research owned a cosmetic and natural foods company, Avacare, Inc., that marketed aloe-based products. Rapidly, Dr. McAnalley found that the fresh gel of the plant facilitated wound healing. Processed gel lost this property in a very short period of time, depending on the temperature at which it was stored.

In the next step of the research, Dr. McAnalley found that it was possible to protect and preserve the healing property of the aloe leaf gel. The desirable activity in aloe gel now had a shelf-life, if processed by the procedure Dr. McAnalley developed and patented. The original cosmetic company was sold and a biotechnical company, Carrington Laboratories, Inc., was created to fund and benefit from the sponsored research. Dr. McAnalley was named Director of Research for Carrington Laboratories, and he assembled a scientific team to isolate and identify the labile material in the gel responsible for the healing activity of aloe. The team eventually determined the active healing principle to be a carbohydrate. The scientific community responded to this finding as heresy. Conventional wisdom was that sugars and starches were only sources of energy.

The molecular structure of the molecule was determined by Drs. McAnalley, Eric Moore, and Alexis Eberendu to be a complex carbohydrate comprised of linked mannose sugars called a polyacetylated mannan (PAM). This uniquely structured PAM molecule ultimately was named acemannan. The controversy among scientists over whether aloe gel is medically useful was determined to be caused by the action of an enzyme naturally present in the leaf gel. This enzyme, amannosidase, digests the PAM to a sugar, specifically mannos-6-phosphate. Once this mannan sugar is destroyed by the enzyme, the biological activity disappears. The molecular structure of this PAM was defined and Carrington filed a composition of matter patent, the strongest patent that can be issued, to protect its research and intellectual property. This type of patent has been applied for and issued in multiple countries with major medical markets.

Prior to the sale of Avacare, products were formulated with aloe gel specially processed and stabilized to protect its biological activity (PAMs) from destruction. This occurred prior to discovering the specific source or nature of the gel's healing properties. Anecdotal reports soon were coming into the company relating to remarkable and unparalleled health benefits obtained by consumers who used the improved gel added to cosmetics and as a result of drinking the company's aloe beverage, Caraloe® .

Among these informal reports came remarkable claims made by eight AIDS patients who did not know one another and lived in four separate states. The AIDS victims stated that the aloe drink eliminated their fever, fatigue, and opportunistic infections. These AIDS patients previously had been unable to work or attend school, but claimed to have returned to normal activity after three to four months of drinking Caraloe® .

At this point, Dr. McAnalley turned to a local Grand Prairie physician, H. Reg McDaniel, M.D., to evaluate the reports from these AIDS patients. Initially, Dr. McDaniel declined and discredited the reports for improvement in the AIDS patients as fanciful and unfounded.

In time, Dr. McAnalley convinced Dr. McDaniel to conduct and/or supervise three AIDS clinical pilot studies. A total of 41 patients were observed and monitored while receiving oral PAM. While these clincial studies were being conducted, Dr. McDaniel, an anatomical and clinical laboratory pathologist, set up a molecular biology and tissue culture laboratory in an empty suite near the Dallas-Fort Worth Medical Center complex. The mission of the new laboratory was to grow cells and viruses and to test sterile PAMs against infectious viral agents. It was shown on a dose-response basis that the PAMs were antiviral against such viruses as herpes, measles, rhinotracheitis, and the HIV-1 (AIDS) virus. Molecular biology procedures confirmed that inhibition of AIDS virus production was induced by the PAMs and that target cells were protected from infection by the retrovirus. It also was demonstrated that if a person's leukocytes (white cells) were harvested and put in culture, they initially were infected readily with an HIV-1 virus challenge in culture chambers. This same person's leukocytes developed resistance to HIV-1 if the donor took oral PAMs prior to white cell harvest from his blood, followed by virus challenge in culture chambers.

During this interval, Robert Carpenter, D.V.M., a research veterinarian, joined the Carrington scientific team. He conducted important animal preclinical studies and organized human clinical toxicity studies required by FDA regulations. He contributed pivotal observations and experimental designs that helped determine how and why PAMs are antiviral and immune system stimulants. In addition, he directed the veterinary approval of PAMs as a vaccine adjuvant and in the treatment of solid tumor cancers in dogs and cats.

Drs. Carpenter, McAnalley, and McDaniel are listed as co-inventors on a series of acemannan use patents that cover over 100 abnormal conditions in man and animals for which PAMs have demonstrated benefit under medical scrutiny in an experimental setting. In addition, over thirty scientific articles and presentations on PAMs have been presented to the medical and scientific community in journals and at major meetings in the United States and Europe by these same three researchers. In response, AIDS experts have been disinterested—or cool at best—to these presentations.

Clinical experimentation with AIDS patients started in December, 1985, with guidance from an FDA regulatory consultant. Following the filing of a treatment protocol with the FDA, 14 AIDS patients were started on oral PAMs by Dr. McDaniel. Within two weeks, symptoms began to improve in all but the most advanced patients. Using a combination of clinical and laboratory criteria at 90 days therapy, a 71% improvement in the group's symptoms was documented.

A second pilot group of 15 AIDS patients were treated in 1986 with oral PAMs by Terry Pulse, M.D., and Dr. McDaniel. A 69% improvement in clinical and laboratory parameters was noted at 90 days therapy. In the 29 patients in the two initial pilot studies, helper lymphocyte (CD4) levels rose from low levels to normal, and some to values more than triple the pre-treatment levels.

The HIV-1 virus was cultured readily from patients' blood prior to treatment but could not be isolated after six weeks of oral PAMs. P-24 core antigen levels for the virus dropped or became negative. Patients gained weight, infections subsided, skin test reactions became responsive, and responding patients (approximately 75%) returned to work or resumed their education.

A third pilot comprised of 26 symptomatic HIV-1 patients was conducted by Terry Watson, D.O., of Dallas, and Dr. McDaniel. In this group, a pre-treatment prediction of how the patients would respond was made from initial laboratory work. Similar clinical responses as those noted in the first two pilots were obtained. An 87% accuracy for predicting who would and would not respond to PAMs was noted. Patients experienced increased levels of CD4 lymphocytes, reduction in P-24 core antigen, and improvement in clinical scoring for patients with a pre-treatment CD4 lymphocyte count of 150/mm³ (a measure of HIV-1 virus damage to the immune system) or greater and a P-24 core antigen (an expression of HIV-1 virus production) of less than 300 picograms. The clinical pilot results were reported to the FDA. In response, as required by FDA regulations and federal law, further clinical experimentation was put on clinical hold in October 1986. These tests resumed in the US in 1989. Carrington has continued to work under rigorous scientific conditions dictated by federal law toward meeting the safety and efficacy requirements necessary for a prescribed use of a drug for the treatment of disease.

An oral presentation and three scientific posters were presented in Jerusalem, Israel, in 1989 at a macrophage-cytokine international conference. Here, the Texans' work came to the attention of Nathan Clumeck, M.D., of Belgium. Dr. Clumeck is the physician who first identified and published a paper on the AIDS clinical syndrome. Based on the prior results, Dr. Clumeck conducted a double-blind, placebo-controlled clinical study with 50 AIDS/ARC patients with oral AZT and PAMs. He confirmed the results obtained in the Texas pilot studies and noted that the toxicity of AZT probably was reduced by PAMs. In 1992, upon reevaluating the condition of the patients treated in Belgium, the only long-term survivors received PAMs during their brief study. All patients receiving a placebo with their AZT had died.

Accumulated data on the extended status of survivors from the clinical studies conducted in Texas by Dr. McDaniel was presented in San Francisco at the 6th International AIDS Conference in 1990. Results of Dr. Clumeck's clinical study were presented, in conjunction with summary information on the three clinical pilot studies done in Texas. This combined information came to the attention of the AIDS Clinical Trials Network for Canada. The Canadians were impressed and offered to conduct a small formal placebo-controlled clinical study on oral PAMs.

The Canadian study was conducted, however, the results were difficult to evaluate. This was due, in part, to the nature of the patient population. Only very advanced AIDS patients with marked immune system viral damage and severe AZT toxicity injury, and who were dying at a predictable rate, were admitted into the study. In spite of the poor clinical status of the patients, as well as the fact that they continued to receive AZT, when the study code was broken, it was found that the rate of deterioration of those patients who received PAMs was slowed, and a few actually experienced improvement in their clinical status and laboratory values. The statistical analysis of the Canadian study patients was not impressive, yet the clinical implications were encouraging.

Patients in the 1986 clinical pilot started by Dr. Pulse were offered a continued supply of oral PAMs in the form of chemically assayed Caraloe® . They also were provided a free annual evaluation. Three patients who have continued on Caraloe® are alive and free of symptoms in the eighth year since they met the CDC standard for having AIDS. They have had no hospitalizations or serious opportunistic infections. Their lymphocyte levels have remained near normal and tests for immune function indicate their defense system has been restored. They are productive and not on welfare. Suicide has been the primary cause of death for this entire study group.

At the Texas A&M College of Veterinary Medicine, important confirmatory state-of-the-art studies in virology and cell biology were conducted by immunologist Ian Tizard, Ph.D. The A&M researchers also found that PAM is a superior systemic vaccine adjuvant that has revolutionized the economics of the chicken broiler industry. Eventually, the Carrington research team found that PAM is taken into a special leukocyte, the macrophage, and this cell is stimulated to release messenger molecules called cytokines (such as interferons, interleukins, prostaglandins, tumor necrosis factor, and stem-cell growth factors). The result is that general host defense and healing is stimulated. PAM also was found to be an immune modulator. Administration of PAM assisted up-regulated host defense when appropriate and down-regulated host reactions when inappropriate, as in allergies, autoimmune disease, and chemical hypersensitivity reactions.

Researchers at Vanderbilt Medical Center, Nashville, Tennessee, discovered that PAMs alter the synthesis of the AIDS virus envelope necessary for attaching to and entering uninfected lymphocytes. Jasbir Kahlon, Ph.D., virologist at the Southern

Research Institute, Birmingham, Alabama, found that PAMs suppress the synthesis of viral messenger RNA in HIV-1 infected leukocytes. These studies demonstrate that a naturally occurring substance extracted from the aloe plant stimulates to maximum activity the normal cellular physiology of defense and wound healing for animals, including humans.

Armed with basic scientific data and results from multiple clinical pilot studies, in 1993 Galen Marshall, M.D., Ph.D., Professor of Immunology and Allergy at the University of Texas Health Science Center in Houston, was granted permission by the FDA to inject sterile, purified PAMs using a multiple ascending protocol into 50 medical students. In this human toxicity study, no liver, bone marrow, or kidney damage or other organ cell toxicity was noted. On the strength of this data, the FDA recently granted Dr. Marshall permission to start injections of PAMs into AIDS patients.

To provide additional research funds for the rapidly expanding and very expensive clinical testing in humans, Dr. McAnalley began direct development of an oral use for PAMs and entered it in the FDA regulatory process. In 1986, Dr. McDaniel had conducted a clinical pilot study for treating ulcerative colitis and Crohn's disease using a relatively crude freeze-dried aloe product formulated in capsules. The results were very encouraging for this poorly managed disease for which there is no known cause, cure, or good treatment.

In 1993-94, a six-center clinical study for treatment of colitis with oral acemannan was conducted with Vanderbilt Medical Center Gastroenterology Department as the primary investigator site. The report on these colitis patients' response to oral PAMs to the FDA has provided the basis to start a Phase II clinical study projected to start in 1995.

The possibility to sell oral PAM capsules for colitis suggested another source of funding to allow Carrington to support the AIDS protocol enmeshed in the regulatory process. Unexpectedly, in June 1994, the FDA gave permission to start the next step in AIDS testing at the UTHSC in Houston under Dr. Marshall's professional direction.

The need for an aloe source below the winter-freeze zone became apparent in 1982 when the aloe fields in the Texas Rio Grand Valley were destroyed and required two years to be replanted and reach maturity. Aloe research at Carrington virtually was suspended during this interval. In anticipation of a future demand for PAMs, Carrington developed an aloe plantation in Costa Rica and built a processing plant to FDA pharmaceutical specifications to freeze-dry the stabilized aloe gel extract. The plant in Costa Rica has significant unused capacity beyond Carrington's wound gel market. This additional capacity will be needed after Carrington receives FDA permission to market the pharmaceutical acemannan. Manapol^{TM} is the patented food grade extract from the aloe leaf that contains a standardized level of PAMs, along with other valuable trace elements found in the gel. The source of Carrington's aloe PAMs is a plantation rich in volcanic ash soils. In that tropical climate, no commercial fertilizer, irrigation, pesticides, or fungicides are used in local fields or surrounding farms. Since the leaves are harvested and the gel extracted and converted to a dry powder on the same day, no stabilizers or preservatives are used or present in Manapol^{TM}. The rapid, patented processing of the fresh aloe prevents any loss or deterioration of the labile PAMs.

Carrington faced practical problems in selling the new product Manapol^{TM}. It is costly to establish and maintain a sales force, there is a time-lag from start-up to the first sale of product, and there would be the necessity for a multimillion dollar advertising campaign to create public awareness and a demand for Manapol^{TM}. Thus, Carrington signed an exclusive contract for Manapol^{TM} distribution and sales with Emprise International, Inc., Grand Prairie, Texas. Emprise is a direct or network sales organization. It is headquartered near the DFW-International Airport.

Drs. McAnalley, Carpenter, and McDaniel joined Emprise at this point to assist Biochemist and Chief Executive Officer Bill Fioretti in formulating Manapol^{TM} into three types of consumer health products. The first group is skin care and skin treatment products that utilize the "functional component" in fresh aloe gel. The second type consists of products that optimize the immune response. My brother's experience is the best testimony to the power of the "live" products.

The third type of products supports hormonal balance and production. Since hormones regulate every cell function in the body, they influence the burning of fat, the building of lean tissue, the healthy impact of both good and bad cholesterol, and in short, the metabolic process of every function of the body. As we age, our natural production and balance of hormones is negatively impacted by the diminishing supply of prohormones, such as pregnenolone and DHEA.

The herb dioscorea has been known for years to contain compounds called plant sterols that have been utilized phamaceutically in the production of progesterone and estrogen. When Fioretti, Carpenter, McAnalley, and McDaniel formulated Manapol™ and dioscorea together, they discovered that this unique combination supplemented prohormone production. This is a major breakthrough in the natural support of endocrine function that works hand in hand with the body's immune system and metabolism.

The anticipation of Manapol™-based products was so great that the first day these new products were available, $22,000 in orders were received by Emprise. Today, just a few months later, sales have exceeded $3 million per month, as more and more people have discovered the availability of Manapol™ in consumer products.

According to Dr. McDaniel, "The patented combination of immune and hormonal support products appears to provide the body with important molecules not found in other foods or supplements, and as a result, we started seeing things happen in people that we never could have predicted." To begin validating some of these results, Emprise initiated a clinical study in January, 1995, through the Health and Medical Foundation in Houston, Texas, under the direction of Dr. Gil Kaats. The following is the initial data reported by Dr. Kaats on this clinical trial.

PRELIMINARY CLININICAL TEST DATA

A total of 200 subjects participated in the clinical study, 100 at the Center for Applied Research in San Antonio, Texas, and 100 at Columbia/HCA's Medical Center Hospital in Houston, Texas. During the first eight weeks, subjects followed the same Optimal Health Plan that participants will be asked to follow in the planned field trials. At the time of this writing, 30% of the subjects (N = 59) had completed their first eight weeks on the plan. The results of the trials revealed that by following the plan, subjects:

- accelerated the loss of excess body fat
- maintained or enhanced muscle tissue
- decreased LDL cholesterol (the harmful cholesterol)
- increased appetite control, decreased food cravings
- improved the following self-reported symptoms:

Headaches	Chronic Tension
Irritable Bowel Syndrome	Lack of Energy
Arthritis	Food Allergies
Premenstrual Syndrome	Overeating
Recurring Sinus Infections	Stomach Pain
Tension Fatigue Syndrome	Back Pain
Recurrent Anxiety	Dizziness
Recurrent Depression	Constipation or Diarrhea
Insomnia	Stomach Gas or Indigestion
Binge Eating	Inability to Concentrate

What particularly is interesting to me is the fact that almost every subject who claimed some symptom reported improvement, whether or not their body composition changed. I also was struck by the diversity of symptoms affected.

The renowned Dr. Joe Glickman, Jr., Editor and Chief of numerous medical publications, recently stated that even though the discovery of antibiotics in the 1940s has been the biggest medical breakthrough in decades, the Carrington aloe discovery might have an even bigger impact. Carrington's discovery and patents for the aloe polyacetylated mannans have created quite a controversy in the aloe industry. Aloe manufacturers have begun to realize that the historical healing benefits of aloe vera now have been scientifically linked to this patented substance. And while this might be bad news to general "over-the-counter" aloe manufacturers, it is great news for consumers who have long awaited aloe products that measure up to the *effectiveness* of *fresh* aloe gel.

The focus and commitment to medical research determines the horizons and the reach of the vision for the future that a bio-pharmaceutical can attain. The mechanisms of action found for aloe polyacetylated mannans by the Carrington research team support the vast health and healing claims that have been made for aloe vera by priests, witch doctors, healers, and grandmothers. The business success that can be achieved through the distribution and use of the scientifically defined active principle in aloe for maintaining good health and to relieve human suffering has been termed another "Texas Gusher." The accomplishments realized already are founded on solid science, originating out of the pharmacology and molecular biology laboratory, followed by application in the research clinic, combined and seasoned with the wisdom of observations made over the eons of past history.

The final chapter in the old mystery and scientific controversy concerning aloe vera health claims might emerge as a revolution in medical science. One may view a new era of health care effected through use of this patented aloe discovery. My brother's story is just one of the thousands of success anecdotes reported through the use of this amazing aloe component.

I particularly am thrilled about the numerous reports on the positive impact these products are making on conditions such as ADD and other childhood disorders that have become too commonplace in our country. And, finally, since aging begins at birth, my hope has returned for the millions of children who are growing up in an environment loaded with industrial toxins that abuse their immune systems and can rob them of their precious health.

Robert M. Siegel, M.D., F.A.A.P.

Dr. Siegel graduated Phi Beta Kappa. He practiced pediatrics in Dallas for 35 years. During that time, he served as Chief of Staff for Children's Hospital and Chief of Pediatric Staff at both St. Paul Hospital and Brookhaven Hospital. Additionally, he was a clinical instructor at Southwestern Medical School and Children's Medical Center. He held staff privileges at RHD Memorial, St. Paul Presbyterian, and Baylor Hospitals. He continues membership in the American Medical Society, Texas Medical Society, Dallas County Medical Society, and the American Academy of Pediatrics.

Dr. Siegel has been the major principal in the start-up of many businesses, including Applied Biogenics Corp. of California and Easy Ware Software Corp. Dr. Siegel, his brother, and a bio-professor, started Dallas Enviro-Health Lab, Inc., and took it public.

In 1984, he retired from his medical practice to work on a series of books. In his research, he identifies a blueprint to human nature. His theory links a unified system of nature—tracing fundamental quantum forces which align physical, biological, and human behaviors. Understanding a grand plan of Nature at work—through natural systems of energy exchange—helps clarify the events of our own everyday personal lives.

About eight years ago, his brother was diagnosed with cancer. His focus turned to immunity research, and he became part of a leading-edge, brainstorming group working on new discoveries of *natural precursor nutrients* (phyto-chemicals). These functional molecules choreograph the inborn natural behaviors of our metabolic, endocrine, and immune systems —which constitute our body's *own* defense against disease and its natural methods of healing. Nature uses key, essential phyto-chemicals to regulate our health and wellness. The ace mannon molecule serves as the precursor for regulating the critical pathways of immunity. Dioscorea regulates DHEA to balance (as needed) our hormonal energies. These basic systems work together in synergy. This new wave of science and nature working together—through "mother molecules"—will open the gateway to our richer health in the 21st Century.

— RESPONSE PAGE —

I read about the great discoveries related to aloe vera and the Manapol™ products in Lindsey Williams' book, *You Can LIVE!*

☐ Please send me a catalog describing Emprise products.

☐ I am interested in becoming an Associate in the distribution of Emprise products. Please send me information.

☐ Please process my order for Emprise products, as follows:

CODE	QTY.	PRODUCT DESCRIPTION	UNIT PRICE	COST
101		MVP™ (90 Cap.)	$39.00	$
111		PLUS™ (90 Cap.)	39.00	
121		SPORT™ (60 Cap.)	35.00	
131		FIRM™ (6 oz.)	39.00	
141		MAN•ALOE™ (60 Cap.)	39.00	
151		PHYT•ALOE™ (60 Cap.)	39.00	
161		NATURALIZER™ (2 oz.)	39.00	
171		EMPRIZONE™ (2 oz.)	39.00	
181		PHYTO•BEARS™ (60/Box)	19.50	
191		EM•PACT™ (150/Box)	39.00	

SUBTOTAL	$
SHIPPING & HANDLING	3.50
TOTAL	$

Thank you!

PLEASE PRINT:

Name _____

Address _____

City/State/Zip _____

Telephone (_____) _____

☐ Payment enclosed with order.
☐ VISA and ☐ MasterCard accepted. Exp. Date_____

No. _____-_____-_____-_____

Auth'd Signature _____

Please make your selection(s) and send to:

PREV-CARE ENTERPRISES, INC.
Dr. Robert M. Siegel
3005 S. Lamar Blvd. D-109-382 • Austin, TX 78704-4785
Attn: S. M. Siegel
TOLL-FREE Order No. 1-800-807-4779 • Fax: (512) 707-9665

Chapter 8

Aromatherapy— The Missing Link in Modern Medicine

By D. Gary Young, N.D., Aromatologist
Creator of Essential Oil Formulas, Food Supplements, and
Skin Care Products

According to the translation of ancient Egyptian hiero-glyphics and Chinese manuscripts, priests and physicians were using oils thousands of years before the time of Christ. There are 188 references to oils in the Bible.

> Moreover the Lord spake unto Moses, saying, Take thou also unto thee principal spices, of pure myrrh ...of sweet cinnamon...of sweet calamus...of cassia...and of oil olive...and thou shalt make it an oil of holy ointment, an ointment compound after the art of the apothecary: it shall be an holy anointing oil. (Exodus 30:22-25)

Some precious oils, such as frankincense, myrrh, rosemary, hyssop, cassia, cinnamon, and spikenard, were used for the anointing and healing of the sick. Biblical prophets recognized the use of essential oils as a protection for their bodies against the ravages of disease. The wise men brought the oils of frank-incense and myrrh to the Christ-child. Clinical research now shows that frankincense oil contains very high immune-stimu-lating properties. The ancient process of oil distillation is a delicate and precise art that almost has been forgotten. Science just now is rediscovering the healing substances that were used in ancient times and beginning to acknowledge their value.

On February 8, 1973, I was injured in a logging accident that paralyzed me for life, according to the medical specialists. After nearly two years of severe pain and depression, I decided to take action and take control of my own life. I began to research and study different methods of alternative healing and started my gradual regeneration. Over a period of two years, I went from the wheelchair to a walker, to crutches, and then to walking, but not without considerable pain. After receiving a master's degree in nutrition and a doctorate in Naturopathy, I opened a clinical family practice in Chula Vista, California, and a research clinic in La Mesa, Mexico, in 1982.

In 1983, I studied the existing research on Tea Tree Oil and incorporated it into my practice for cuts, bruises, burns, pain, etc. However, after a year, I was very disappointed with the poor results. I read other research and information on essential oils but never really became excited until I was invited to attend a medical seminar being held at the Medical University in Geneva, Switzerland. This seminar was taught by medical doctors Jean Claude Lapraz and Paul Duraffourd on respiratory disease and essential oils. I returned to my clinic with 13 oils and great anticipation. The research was incredible, as I discovered how the oils could increase cellular oxygen and promote immune function.

Primarily, I was concerned with helping my patients and had not considered how I might benefit from the oils personally. After 13 years, I still suffered with pain and had great limitations, being able to walk only short distances. One morning, awakening with intense pain, the thought came to me to use the oils on myself. Within three days, I was walking without pain; one week later, I was jogging for the first time in 13 years. In November of 1986, I entered a half-marathon and finished 60th out of 970 participants.

As one might well understand, this propelled me with even

greater speed and intensity into learning and uncovering the mysteries of essential oils.

ANCIENT AROMAS

Aroma is the oldest means of reaching and influencing man's deepest instincts. When we examine creation, we find that everything from dust to man has an odor. Ancient physicians diagnosed disease by the individual's odor.

The famous French detective Vidocq states, "If I am in a crowd of over 1,000 people, I can single out every violator of the moral law by the smell." He stated that every area of criminal activity has its own odor, and he could identify each one.

In 1817, the Ebers Papyrus was discovered. It was over 870 feet long and referred to as a medicinal scroll. It dated back to 1500 B.C. and mentioned over 800 different formulations of herbal prescriptions and remedies. Other scrolls indicate that the Egyptians had a very high success rate in the treating of 81 different diseases. They made many mixtures of myrrh oil and honey. Myrrh still is recognized for its ability to help with infections of the skin and throat and to regenerate skin tissue. Myrrh was used for embalming because of its effectiveness in preventing bacteria growth.

In about the 8th Century, the Arabs, as both merchants and warriors, spread the remedies from Asia Minor to the Middle East and worked on improving the method of extracting essential oils.

The ancient Egyptians first discovered the oils and aromatic uses of oils for medicine long before the raw plant was examined and incorporated into their field of medicine.

It is easy to look back into history and see that essential oils are the oldest form of medicine known to man. The Chinese people became aware of aromatics, and documents recorded by the Emperor Kiwang-ti indicate the use of opium, pomegranate, rhubarb, and aromatic substances in the Chinese sanskrit of 2000 B.C. The Greeks elaborated on the use of essential oils to include hair, skin, and body massage for the feet, jaws, joints, and perhaps in the preventing of arthritic-type symptoms. The Romans also played an important role in the history of essential oils. They used essential oils and perfumes with virtually everything, and particularly with the care of their bodies.

Throughout the Old Testament and up to the time of Christ, we read about the value of oils. What happened to these oils after Christ? Perhaps during the Middle Ages and the burning of the libraries in Alexandria much of this knowledge was lost, and only through the cosmetic and perfume industry did this incredible science begin to resurface. With the use of modern technology in the field of medical science and research and the translation of ancient writings, we will be able to rediscover these healing substances as they were meant for us to use by our Creator.

WHAT IS AROMATHERAPY? THE SCIENCE OF ESSENTIAL OILS

Aromatherapy is a phrase coined by Dr. René-Maurice Gattefossé, a French cosmetic chemist, in 1920. He had a laboratory accident and received third degree burns on his hand and forearm. He saw that his colleague had just brought in a container from the cooler. Thinking it was water, he plunged his arm into the vat to cool it. However, it was lavender oil. To his surprise, the burning slowly decreased and then stopped within a few moments. Over a period of time, with the continual application of lavender oil, the burn healed completely without a trace of a scar. Dr. Gattefossé became very excited with the potential healing properties contained in aromatic substances. He started to analyze the essential oil of lavender and discovered that it contained many properties referred to as chemical constituents or chemical properties.

As a result, Dr. Gattefossé determined that essential oils— the aromatic substances in flowers, trees, shrubs, herbs, bushes, roots, seeds, leaves, stems, and flowering petals—contained a semi-oily resin with tremendous healing properties. Thus, the ancient art of Aromatherapy began its reentry into the modern world.

Dr. Gattefossé shared his experience with his colleague, Dr. Jean Valnet, a medical doctor in Paris, France. During World War II, while serving as a medical physician in the French Army at the China Wall, Valnet ran out of antibiotics and other medications that customarily were being used. He reverted to using essential oils. To his amazement, the essential oils had a powerful effect in stopping and reducing infection. He was able to save many of the soldiers who otherwise would have died, even with antibiotics.

Dr. Paul Belaiche and Dr. Jean Claude Lapraz picked up on Dr. Valnet's work in the early 1960's, conducting laboratory research and opening a practice using essential oils. They discovered that essential oils contain antiviral, antibacterial, antifungal, and antiseptic properties, as well as being powerful oxygenators with the ability to act as a catalyst in the delivery of nutrients into the cells. These doctors have contributed greatly to the research by writing manuscripts, papers, and books on the treatment of infectious disease with oils.

The wholeness and complexity of Aromatherapy gives it the potential to do what it does. If you take a geranium plant and tear the leaf or the stem, a clear liquid will appear. This liquid is a very subtle and volatile essence that exudes from the damaged tissues of the leaf. So it is with the human body. With a cut or scrape, we see a flow of blood from that opening in the skin.

One significant difference between the blood and the plant liquid is the color. In the resin or oil being released from the plant, we find trace elements of nutrients, hormones, enzymes, vitamins, minerals, antibodies, and antifungal, antibacterial, anti-infectious, antiseptic, and immune-stimulating properties. One other key agent found present in that resin—which is so important for sustaining and regenerating—is **oxygen**. Oxygen molecules are found within the chemical elements of the resin, such as alcohols, phenols, esters, sesquiterpenes, terpinols, etc., which together create an essential oil.

The plant releases the oil in order to clean the break, kill bacteria, and start the regeneration process. When blood is released because of broken skin, it is for the same purpose: to clean the wound, kill the bacteria, prevent infection, and begin the healing and regeneration process. A simple comparison of the plant with the human body shows us a precise similarity, as both the oil and the blood are the transporters of the fundamental nutrients necessary to feed and nurture the cells. *Essential oils have been found to help increase oxygen because they are antioxidants.* They contain oxygenating molecules and, therefore, have the ability to increase cellular oxygen, thus giving more support to the immune system. It has been said that anyone who uses essential oils on a continuous basis has a stronger immune system, and research has confirmed their immune-stimulating properties, whether they are inhaled or rubbed on the body topically. Even those who contract a cold or flu recover 70% faster using essential oils.

It is believed that when essential oils are diffused in the home, they have the ability to increase the atmospheric oxygen, as they release oxygenating molecules into the atmosphere. Oils increase ozone and negative ions in the home, which inhibit bacteria growth. This prevents the growth of mold and destroys existing odors from mold, cigarettes, animals, etc. Essential oils have the electrical magnetic attraction to fracture the molecular chain of chemicals and take them out of the air, rendering them nontoxic to the body. Scientists in Europe have found that essential oils will bond to metallics and chemicals and carry them out of the body, working as a natural chelator. These are all wonderful attributes of essential oils. They remove dust particles out of the air and, *when diffused in the home, can be the greatest air filtration system in the world.*

Essential oils can be extracted from different parts of the plant or tree. It is even possible for different oils to be extracted from the same tree. For example, from the orange tree the orange peel can be pressed for orange oil, the leaves and twigs distilled for pettigrain oil, and the orange blossoms for neroli oil. One tree can produce three different types of oils that are beneficial or therapeutic in three or more different ways.

Today, there are about 200 different types of oils being distilled, with several thousand chemical constituents and aromatic molecules which have been identified and registered. These aromatic substances and compounds within the oils will alter and change, based on weather conditions, climate, temperatures, and distillation factors. Today, 98% of essential oils are used in the perfume and cosmetic industry. In 1991, only ½% was used in Aromatherapy. In 1993, production for therapeutic and medicinal purposes increased to 2½%.

Essential oils have been recognized for their ability to decrease the viscosity of the blood and increase the velocity, thus *increasing cellular oxygen.* The greater the circulation of the blood, the greater the oxygenation to the tissue. Essential oils are recognized as being the greatest substances for increasing cellular oxygen through their normal function. When applied to the body by rubbing on the feet, essential oils will travel throughout the body and saturate every cell, including the hair, within 20 minutes.

It has been discovered that one of the causes of disease in both the plant and the human body is the inability of nutrients to penetrate the cell wall, causing cell deterioration, which leads to cell mutation, creating a host for bacteria and disease. One of the incredible aspects of the oils is their ability to penetrate and carry nutrients *through* the cell wall to the cell nucleus.

The textbook, *L'aromatherapie exactement,* gives us the description, definition, and prescribing application by doctors in Europe for 86 different essential oils, along with their properties responsible for antiviral, antibacterial, antifungal, anti-infectious, and immune-stimulating activities.

In 1990, I met Jean-Noël Landel, with whom I became partners in a research farm in southern France. We started out with 12 acres, which now has increased to 320. Over the past three years, I have studied at Cairo University under the direction of Dr. Radwan Farag, who is the head of the biochemistry department. Dr. Farag documented the oxygenating molecule activity in essential oils and was responsible for the discovery of their antioxidant and antimicrobial activity.

Aromatherapy is a simple term used to cover a very broad subject and an incredible field that we just now are beginning to explore—a field which I believe may well have a great impact on the well-being of mankind and life on this planet.

Aromatherapy means to treat with aroma through inhalation. As the aroma of the oils passes through the nasal passage, it stimulates the genes along the nose that trigger a response of the neurons that dangle in the sinus cavity from the olfactory bulb. The neurons pick up the oil molecules and the electrical signal and transmit them through the olfactory nerve to the gland called the amygdala, which controls the senses of the body. Dr. Joseph LaDoux of the New York Medical Center has stated that the amygdala is responsible for memory and the processing of both positive and negative emotions. The response to aroma has been proven to be as quick as one to three seconds.

Fragrance is one of man's greatest enjoyments. Fragrance triggers memories of past experiences. The fragrance wafting through the air on a cool summer evening might remind us of a family outing in the park, or the smell of cinnamon rolls might remind us of the aroma we could smell while walking home from school. Fragrance creates a feeling of security, grounding, and well-being.

HOW DO ESSENTIAL OILS WORK? OIL CHEMISTRY AND CONSTITUENTS

Essential oils are chemically very heterogenic, meaning they are very diverse in their effect and have different actions, unlike synthetic chemicals which have basically one action. For example, lavender has been used for burns, insect bites, headaches, PMS, insomnia, stress, etc.

Plants in nature are chemical factories. They take in the elements of the sun and earth, light and darkness—individually—to receive the energy from both, converting them into molecules, carbohydrates, proteins, and fats. These are the crude fuels which are broken down to produce ATP (adenosine triphosphate), which is a high-octane fuel in the body.

Many scientific experiments have shown that essential oils can travel with relative speed when inhaled or applied through massage. The molecules of essential oils are so microscopic that they can penetrate the fatty layers of the skin. The liquid solubility of essential oils allows them to travel transcellularly or directly through the cells. Their penetrating ability through the fatty tissue layers into the interstitial fluids may explain why essential oils enhance circulation and why massage with oils can be so beneficial.

Generally, the immune system can be improved greatly by increasing the velocity (or movement) of the blood and decreasing the viscosity (or thickness) of the blood. This will enhance circulation, which is vital to good health, as it affects the function of every cell and organ, including the brain.

Essential oils are comprised of chemistry groups, as well as individual chemistry elements. Some of the primary elements responsible for the function of essential oils are *hydrogen, carbon, and oxygen*. Most of the more obvious effects of essential oils can be attributed to such properties as oxygen-containing molecules, such as sesquiterpenes, phenols, ketones, alcohols, and aldehydes.

Many of the aromatic constituents found in essential oils are derived from phenylpropanes. These are the precursors of amino acids, which link together to convert nutrients to proteins, which are the building blocks of the human body. Terpeneols are another group of chemical constituents which are created from a single coenzyme A which in the human organism plays a crucial role in the production of vitamins, enzymes, and their conversion to energy. The essential oil constituents found in various oils, such as rosemary, peppermint, clove, cinnamon, melissa, oregano, and thyme, have the ability to increase the production of ATP. They also *increase oxygen absorption within the cells* and permit more efficient utilization of oxygen from other sources, such as food and water.

Essential oils have many different chemical components in their various molecular structures. Aldehydes are anti-infectious, sedative, and calming to the nervous system. They are found predominantly in lavender and chamomile oils. Eugenol is antiseptic and stimulating and is found in cinnamon and clove oils. Ketones, found in lavender, hyssop, and patchouly oils, stimulate cell regeneration, liquify mucus and are helpful with dry asthma, colds, and flu. Phenols are antiseptic and kill bacteria and viruses and are found in oregano and thyme oil. Sesquiterpenes, which are predominantly in frankincense and sandalwood, are anti-inflammatory and work as liver and gland stimulants. They were found in 1994 to go beyond the brain blood barrier, increasing oxygen around the pineal and pituitary glands. Terpene alcohols, found in juniper and citrus, are antibacterial and work as diuretics and decongestants. In 1985, Dr. Jean C. Lapraz said he *couldn't find bacteria or viruses that could live in the presence of the essential oils of cinnamon or oregano.* He found many other oils displaying the same qualities. This is very significant, as today we are faced with life-threatening viruses that seemingly are drug-resistant. We are finding incredible microbial mutations that are beginning to create a panic in various parts of the world, and understandably so.

SPECIFIC FORMULATIONS

I always marvel at the ease of seeing pain diminish in seconds, without even touching the area that is hurt or injured. Bone pain can be unbearably painful and is very difficult to relieve. Yet, simple formulas like **Pane Away** and **Relieve It** have helped thousands of people find pain relief. Pane Away contains an oil called helichrysum, which has topical anesthesia-like action and is a very powerful anti-inflammatory. Relieve It contains spruce, which carries the constituent methyl salicylate that works similar to cortizone. These two blends will take away 75-90% of bone and tissue pain in a matter of minutes and can be used singularly or alternately.

The immune system is another important area we want to examine, especially with the tremendous weakness and continual degeneration caused by the chemicals we ingest, our polluted water and air, our denatured food, and our hectic lifestyles. I saw a tremendous need in this area, so I created an oil formula called **ImmuPower** to help give us some support and protection. This formula contains the oils of ravensara, oregano, thyme, mountain savory, clove, and black cumin, which all are antiviral and antifungal. Oregano, frankincense, clove, and cistus are immune stimulators. Frankincense and clove are antitumoral and anticancerous. The action of the oils in this formula all have been documented by medical doctors and scientists in Europe and published in Dr. Daniel Pénoël's medical text on Aroma-therapy. *Boswellis Carterii* is the botanical name for frankincense (p. 328) and *Origanum compactum* is for oregano (p. 383).

I was amazed when I had my own experience. Shortly after making this formula, I developed a serious throat infection. I didn't pay any attention to it until two days later, when I realized that my sore throat was getting worse, and I was running a fever over 103 °F. My wife rubbed ImmuPower all over my throat and up my spine, and within 30 seconds the fever broke. At the same time, my throat opened up and I felt energy returning to my body. The next morning, it was as though nothing ever had been wrong. I continue to marvel at every new experience and the wonders of essential oils.

FREQUENCY OF ESSENTIAL OILS

Frequency is defined as a measurable rate of electrical energy that is constant between any two points. Everything has an electrical frequency, and what an incredible discovery it was for me to learn that essential oils contain a frequency that is several times greater than the frequency of herbs and foods.

Robert O. Becker, M.D., author of *The Body Electric,* validates the electrical frequency of the human body.

Richard Restick, M.D., one of the leading neurologists in Washington, D.C., and author of *The Brain Has a Mind of Its Own,* talks about the electrical circuitry of the brain and body.

Dr. Royal Raymond Rife developed a "frequency generator" in the early 1920's. With it, he found that certain frequencies could destroy a cancer cell or a virus. He found that certain frequencies could prevent the development of disease and others would destroy disease. Although he now is deceased, he left a legacy of incredible work in the field of frequency and its importance in the human body.

Nikola Tesla said that if you could eliminate certain outside frequencies that interfered in our bodies, we would have greater resistance to disease.

Bjorn Nordenstrom, a radiologist of Stockholm, Sweden, and author of *Biologically Closed Circuits,* discovered in the early 1980's that by putting an electrode inside a tumor and running a milliamp DC current through the electrode, he could dissolve the cancerous tumor and stop its growth. He found that the human body had electropositive and electronegative energy fields.

When we talk about frequency, we may become confused, knowing that light bulbs, television, telephones, electric ranges, refrigerators, dishwashers, toasters, microwaves (heaven forbid), blenders, trash compactors, garbage disposals, clocks, electric blankets, water beds, vibrating chairs, hair dryers, curling irons, computers, fax machines, etc., all have a frequency range around 60 hertz. What we must realize is that there are different kinds of frequencies: incoherent and coherent, chaotic and harmonic, direct current (DC) and alternating current (AC). Electrical lights, appliances, and most man-made devices, have AC incoherent chaotic frequencies. Man, herbs, plant life, essential oils—those things created by God—operate with a DC-like current that has a coherent, harmonic frequency when healthy and in balance. It is like a grand piano that, when tuned correctly, has perfect harmonics and sound; but let one string be out of harmonic balance, and the sound is irritating and "sick."

For a number of years during my clinical practice, I researched the use of electrical energy for the purpose of reversing the disease process. I kept feeling that there had to be a more natural way of increasing a person's electrical frequency, which led to the discovery of the electrical frequency of oils.

One of the things that I noticed with my patients, when they first started to use the oils, was that they felt better emotionally. It seemed that just through simple inhalation of an oil, within seconds congestion would begin to loosen. Certain oils applied on location would decrease pain 50-80% within one to three minutes. Some even experienced a decrease in pain within seconds. I could not have thought that an oil applied to the bottom of the feet could travel to the neck and reduce pain by 70% within one minute. As I saw this happen over and over, I started to realize that there had to be other aspects and elements in the oils which had to be researched.

In 1992, the discovery was made that essential oils have a bioelectrical frequency measurable in hertz, megahertz, and kilohertz, which was substantially higher than anything tested up to this time. Bruce Tainio, of Tainio Technology, an independent division of Eastern State University in Cheny, Washington, was trying to find ways to clean up contaminated water and soil that had been destroyed by heavy chemical saturation. He always had been fascinated with energy and set out to find a machine that would analyze the energies of the soil, water, and plants. He finally decided that he would have to build this machine; so with several other electrical engineers, he built the first frequency monitor in the world. He worked for four years, making alterations and perfecting it until it could be proven to be 100% accurate.

When Bruce Tainio and I began our conversations about frequency, Bruce offered to test the oils for their electrical frequency. I had tested the oils with other instruments and machines, but they were not 100% accurate, therefore not accepted as a valid test. Bruce told me that the machine he had built was certified as 100% accurate and was being used in the agricultural field. That began the great discovery of the electrical frequency of essential oils and the first time in the world that the oils actually had been tested and documented.

Young Living and Tainio Technology were the discoverers of this great work. We determined that the average frequency of the human body during the daytime is between 62-68 hertz (Hz). The brain frequency from 6:00 a.m. to 5:00 p.m. is between 72-78 Hz. Sometimes the frequency will be higher (even up to 80 Hz) with people who are studying for exams or using their minds a lot. Research has shown that if the frequency of the right and left brain lobes varied more than 3 Hz, a headache would begin. If the frequency varied more than 10 Hz, a substantial or migraine-type headache would develop. I made an oil formula called **My-Grain**, containing such oils as helichrysum, chamomile, and lavender, whereby through simple inhalation the frequency in the head could be balanced and the headache reduced in a few seconds. With the oils of cardamon, rosemary, basil, and peppermint, I made a formula called **Clarity** to help increase memory and mental accuracy.

The normal frequency range of the human body is between 62-68 Hz, but if it drops below that, the individual becomes a victim for illness because the immune system will start to shut down. Cold symptoms appear at 58 Hz, flu symptoms at 57 Hz, candida at 55 Hz, epstein bar at 52 Hz, cancer at 42 Hz. There is much research yet to be done, but we are finding that these frequencies coincide 98% of the time with those we have already tested.

If we can keep the body frequency high enough, in addition to keeping it well oxygenated, we will be free of disease.

Measuring in hertz, we found that processed/canned food had a zero Hz frequency, fresh produce had up to 15 Hz, dried herbs from 12-22 Hz, and fresh herbs from 20-27 Hz. Essential oils started at 52 Hz and went as high as 320 Hz, which is the frequency of rose oil. A healthy body, from head to foot, typically has a frequency ranging from 62 to 78 Hz, while disease begins at 58 Hz.

Clinical research shows that essential oils have the highest frequency of any substance known to man, creating an environment in which disease—bacteria, virus, fungus, etc.—cannot live. I believe that the chemistry and frequencies of essential oils have the ability to help man maintain an optimal frequency to the extent that disease cannot exist.

THE ANCIENT ART OF DISTILLATION & THE MODERN TECHNIQUE OF ADULTERATION

During the Neolithic period, it was discovered that fatty oils could be extracted from the olive tree through the process of pressing. These oils were used to protect the skin from the sun, massaged into the hair to keep it from becoming dry and brittle, and used for curing and tanning hides for making clothing. The oils also were used for cooking and bathing.

Once in awhile, individuals using an essential oil for the first time will report that they broke out with a rash or had an allergic reaction. Many reactions are just the body's chemical sensitivity kicking in and saying, "Protect me!" However, when I worked with people with severe allergies, even universal reactors—once they understood that pure essential oils actually detoxify and help reestablish cellular balance—they would calm down and realize that they, in fact, *were not* having a reaction. It's amazing to see how we in America have become so sensitive to things around us, yet at the same time are so desensitized to the things that are killing us, causing allergies, depressing the immune system, creating a weakness for diseases such as candida, epstein bar, chronic fatigue syndrome, hypoglycemia, and universal reactor symptoms, as well as other chemically sensitive problems. It just goes from level one to level six, manifesting different symptoms. Even though doctors are diagnosing us with candida or allergies, many times it is really nothing more than an exaggerated condition of hypoglycemia going through its various stages of mutation.

As I was doing research with a clinically controlled group, it was interesting to see that when people were treated for hypoglycemia, their candida symptoms went away, their epstein bar virus disappeared, and chronic fatigue, allergy, and universal reactor symptoms all seemed to diminish substantially, and even disappear. Based on these findings, it was hard for me to believe that we *really have* all these diseases with which we are diagnosed We must realize that germs and bacteria mutate, as well as viruses, which is why we can go from one symptom to another with the same disease.

Because the sense of smell is so incredible, it is important to understand why we have these sensitivities and reactions. Let's go back to the ancient days of distillation. The most common way of extracting oils from plants, trees, shrubs, flowers, and herbs is through distillation. This is done by sending steam into a chamber that holds the raw product. As the steam rises, it stimulates the oil membranes in the plant, causing them to open, thereby releasing the oil molecule that has a microfine membrane around it. This membrane is there to protect the oil from being fractured while it is released. In nature, as the evening cools, the oil comes closer to the surface. As the day begins, the sun's warmth causes this membrane to open and release the oil into the atmosphere. This is when we start to feel and smell a change in the atmosphere. This is why it is so incredible to walk in the garden or forest in the early morning and feel the increased ozone and negative ions, as well as the oxygenating molecules that have been released at sun-up along with the intense fragrance.

When we look at releasing the oil so that it will retain its medicinal properties for the benefits we desire, we need to discover how we can release the oil in a way similar to that of nature. Vertical steam distillation gives us the greatest potential of protecting that oil and maintaining its integrity in order to render its therapeutic benefits for fragrance and balancing the body. This must work on the areas in the brain that are connected to the limbic system, which affects emotional trauma release, appeases anxiety, and helps overcome depression. In ancient distillation, low pressure (5 lb. or under) and low temperature were extremely important.

Temperature has a very distinct effect on the oils. At certain temperatures, the oil fragrance, as well as the chemical constituents, can be changed. High pressures and high temperatures seem to cause a harshness in the oil, and even the oil pH and the electropositive and electronegative balance are affected greatly.

Some large oil producers are resorting to devious practices to promote and sell oil for a cheaper price. In America, we do not understand oil chemistry nor how to test for quality. A chromatograph, which costs $200,000-$300,000, is a machine that tests the chemical constituents, their percentages, and the range of activity that helps determine their quality. Throughout the world, there are a select few who are trained to smell. This trained individual is called a "Nose." It takes 21 years to become certified and is one of the highest paid professions in the world. This individual can identify toxic constituents within an oil that have caused the adulteration.

Most of the lavender oil sold in America today is lavendin, which is grown and distilled in either China or Russia. The oil production in both locations tests high in nitrates from radioactive fallout. They bring it into France, cut it with synthetic linolol acetate to improve the fragrance, add propylene glycol or SD 40, which is a solvent that has no smell and increases the volume, and then sell it in the United States as lavender oil. We in America don't know the difference and are happy to buy it for $5-$7 a half ounce in health food stores, beauty salons, grocery and department stores, and through mail order.

Frankincense is another example of an adulterated oil. I've seen frankincense sold as low as $25 per ounce. However, this was frankincense distilled with alcohol. The frankincense resin or gum that is sold in Somalia costs $30,000-$35,000 per ton. Many use these cut, synthetic, and adulterated oils (which may cause rashes, burns, or other irritations), then wonder why they don't get the benefit they were told to expect—then they arrive at the conclusion that the benefits of essential oils were highly overrated and that they really don't have very much value.

There are first, second, third, and fourth stages of distillation, with each one becoming weaker, to which synthetic fragrance constituents are added and sold to the unsuspecting public. Many people have jumped on the bandwagon because of the money-making potential that they see in essential oils. They buy cheap oils, rebottle them, label them as 100% pure essential oils, and market them without ever knowing the source of their origin or who was responsible for their distillation.

At the Young Living Research Farm in Idaho, where I have built four different distillers and the only stainless steel vertical steam distiller in North America, we can control our operation to produce the highest possible quality oil. After building the first two, I invented a steam decompression chamber and manifold that delivers the steam at zero pounds of pressure to the chambers. We were very specific in choosing the land, which had never had chemicals on it and hasn't to this day. All our growing and production is strictly organic. Our farms in Utah, France, Egypt, and Inner Mongolia, China, are also organic. Young Living is now supervising the distillation of a large percentage of the oils that we sell, because of the high level of adulteration and inferior quality of oils that are produced around the world. We begin with the seed and take it all the way through the harvest, distillation, formulating, packaging, and marketing. This way, we know what we have and can stand behind the production and the quality.

There are many people in America who, after a weekend

course, call themselves "Aromatherapists." They know absolutely nothing about oil chemistry and the very specific ways in which oils need to be formulated in order to maintain a harmonic synergistic action in oil formulations and products formulated with essential oils. So we have people who take a class or listen to a lecture and say, "Oh, there's nothing to this." They go and buy oils, mix them, and create their own blends. This is fine if it is *only* for fragrance and perfume; but when making oil formulas for a specific therapeutic action, you can alter and change the chemistry action and totally neutralize the effect you are seeking if you don't understand the chemistry. This is another reason I spent 10 years in Europe studying in the universities, laboratories, hospitals, museums, and libraries, traveling to distilleries, farms, and essential oil companies, and any place where I thought I could learn and do research in my desire to have as much knowledge as possible in my quest to help bring this ancient science back to the world. My worldwide research is ongoing, as I continue to seek new (or ancient) ways to produce the finest essential oils possible.

Many books sold on essential oils in America are of grave concern to me. The people who are *doing* the actual work and teaching have not taken the time to write and publish books. The journalists who write the books are not the ones doing the research. Many of the books sold in America have little validity in the things they say and the claims they make. Read them with caution, with an open mind, *and with the understanding that a lot of what you read is not true.* One popular book in America is written by a woman claiming to be a medical doctor. However, she bought her degree in Sri Lanka for $1,000, and most of her material has been plagiarized from doctors and researchers involved in doing this great work. I do, however, recommend the books written by Jean Valnet, M.D., Marguerite Maury, Daniele Ryman, and Shirley Price.

EMOTIONS & THE ESSENTIAL OIL CONNECTION

The cure of the part should not be attempted without treatment of the whole, and also no attempt should be made to cure the body without the soul, and therefore if the head and body are to be well you must begin by curing the mind: that is the first thing. . . .

*For this is the great error of our day in the treatment
of the human body, that physicians separate the soul
from the body.* (Plato, Chronicles 156 e)

Frankincense is mentioned approximately 52 times in the Bible,
of which 32 times it is referred to as incense. The Greek/ Hebrew
translation of incense means frankincense. Frankincense has
been recognized since ancient times as the holy anointing oil.
One of the reasons that it obtained this legendary title is because
the ancient priests and physicians found they could rub it on
the sick people and they would get well almost immediately.

Modern science now shows us that *frankincense has the ability
to increase the oxygen around the pineal and pituitary glands.*
Frankincense has been found to help alleviate manic depressive
symptoms. Because it is high in sesquiterpene activity, it has the
ability to work as an immune stimulant. It also contains anticarcinogenic properties and is now being studied for its efficacy
in the possible treatment of various cancers.

The emotional benefits of essential oils were another amazing
aspect which I discovered quite by accident. This was an area
that was rarely mentioned in my travels around the world. Almost
everyone I asked—hoping to learn more about the emotional
connection to oils—would laugh at the idea. However, when I
was testing different oils in the clinic for antiallergy effects (such
as lavender and Roman chamomile), I noticed that the patients
became rather complacent, relaxed, and calm. These were the
same people who either were depressed or hyperactive just an
hour earlier.

Subsequently, I developed three formulations to assist with
emotional difficulties. They are called **Inspiration, Release,** and
Joy.

ESSENTIAL OILS AS FLAVORING IN FOOD & VITAMIN SUPPLEMENTATION

I wouldn't be surprised to find that 80% or more of the
American population is constipated. Most people seem to have
digestive problems such as gas, bloating, indigestion, morning
sickness, etc. Now, some just use a little of the essential oil
formula, **Di-Tone,** which contains peppermint oil, rub it on their
stomachs, and are surprised that their symptoms go away almost

immediately. It is wonderful to know that we don't have to ingest the oils for them to work. However, when used as a food additive, they increase the absorption of the nutrients. I discovered in clinical practice, while doing bacteriology studies with the blood, that there was an incredible amount of food bacteria in the blood serum because (1) it didn't digest, and (2) it couldn't get through the cell wall because of low oxygen levels. It was determined that if we put essential oils in the food products, we wouldn't find any undigested food bacteria in the blood. Through these studies, I discovered several things were happening:

1. The food digested better. Essential oils, like rosemary, aniseed, juniper, peppermint, and tarragon, aided in digestive enzyme secretion.
2. Essential oils digested and prevented unfriendly bacteria growth.
3. Essential oils acted as a catalyst and were soluble with the lipids in the membranes. Therefore, they went directly inside the cell and piggy-backed nutrients of similar harmonic frequency and value in the cell at the same time.
4. The oxygenating molecules increased cell metabolism and helped in balancing the pH of the cell for increased nutritional intake of the food in the body.
5. Because various oils contain phenylpropanes, the precursor of amino acids, they helped strengthen all body functions.

My next challenge, which took two-and-a-half years to discover, was to find a method of adding the oils to my herbal food supplements. One of the reasons I began to formulate supplements myself was because in my clinic I would see patients passing *whole* herbs, vitamin tablets, and capsules during their colonics (colon irrigating), after having ingested them 6 to 12 days prior to their colonics.

Essential oils contain all the healing nutrients, oxygenating molecules, amino acid precursors, coenzyme-A factors, trace amounts of minerals, enzymes, vitamins, hormones, etc., in a concentrated form when distilled. However, today, man cuts the herbs and dehydrates them, destroying 90% of the healing nutrients and the oxygen (which delivers the nutrients to the cells). Then we wonder why herbs don't have the same potency they used to have. If you take the blood out of the human body, you have a corpse. If you take the oil out of the plant, you have only the fiber, devoid of the healing life-force.

When I started to understand this, it seemed to me that we needed that life-force back in the plant, so I started experimenting with oils as a food additive and flavoring agent. This was the most revolutionary development in the health food industry.

VitaGreen, the first food product with essential oils, was formulated to bring the blood back to an alkalinity pH because disease cannot develop in an alkaline, free-flowing blood stream. Barley grass juice is the highest alkaline food we have. Alfalfa sprouts are 52% alkaline protein. Spirulina, Norwegian kelp, bee pollen, amino acids, and essential oils were formulated during my clinical practice to help those who could not digest food and to balance blood sugar and for those who had a greater need for more pre-digested alkaline protein. Before I put the oils in **VitaGreen,** my patients only had 42% blood absorption in 24 hours. After I put the oils in this supplement, the blood absorption increased to 64% in 30 minutes and 86% in one hour. This started to make amazing changes in my patients, and we saw immune function "kick in" from **VitaGreen** alone. I ascertained this was because it was the first nutrition that had penetrated the cell wall in quite some time.

When you feed the body properly, the body can heal itself. However, I have seen people supposedly eating well and dying from disease because they could not get the nutrition into the cell because the food was devoid of its natural nutritional delivery agent. The oils are nature's most natural catalyst and delivery agent.

The next formulas into which I put the oils were **ComforTone** and **I.C.P.** I formulated them to assist in cleansing the intestinal tract of toxic debris and parasites, which are a host for many diseases. Parasites are very difficult to get rid of, and I didn't realize this until I assisted in the operating room with some of my patients who required surgery. It was there that I witnessed the grotesque sight of a human body eaten alive by worms. The first time I saw this, the patient had been eating herbs, garlic, and pumpkin seeds for seven years because Dr. Bernard Jensen, D.C., had diagnosed her with parasites, and he was right. We literally removed over four quarts of worms from her abdomen, many the size of my little finger. This motivated me to make these two formulas, each containing seven oils. Patchouly, for example, aids in the digestion of toxic waste. Tarragon, ginger, and mugwort help the garlic oil to be absorbed into the intestinal lining, penetrating the parasite pockets or nests. Rosemary kills fungus and aids in digestive secretion. Peppermint is antiparasitic, soothes an inflamed colon, and reduces fever. After adding the oils, patients started passing parasites within 12-13 hours. We also have had reports that **ComforTone** and **I.C.P.** bring about the same results in animals.

Body Balance was a formula I made to feed my patients who could not eat solid food. It was difficult to nutritionally support the body on liquids alone, so development of **Body Balance** required great study and selection of the right nutrients. Many people avoided the soy isolate because they claimed it was not digestible; therefore, many health food manufacturers threw it out. However, the pure soy isolate is 92% pure protein. We found that by fractionating the isolate, it was easier to digest. I then added more enzymes, using grade A fructose as a sweetener with grapefruit oil, giving **Body Balance** a great flavor. Five other citrus oils were added, which have been found to help decongest the lymphatic system and increase leukocyte production. Pure fructose is the only sweetener that is really safe for diabetics, doesn't ferment in the stomach, and also converts to pure protein glucose sugar.

It was easy to monitor the progress of a patient and the effectiveness of the formulas when they were in-house, in a clinical environment for two to six weeks. If a formula didn't appear to be working, I could change it until it did work. My clinical practice gave me the great foundation for the development of this important work in which I am now engaged.

Subsequently, I researched putting together programs so people could get benefits at home. The first program formulated for individual use at home now is called **The Cleansing Trio**. This program contains **ComforTone**, **I.C.P.**, and **Megazyme**. **Megazyme** is an enzyme complex to aid in the digestion of toxic material, as well as help with the cleansing and promotion of better assimilation. The first step to good health is cleansing the body, then feeding it good nutrients.

The second program is called **The Body Balancing Trio**, which contains **VitaGreen**, **Body Balance**, and **Master Formula His and Hers**. **Body Balance** is great in water alone, but one also can add different oils for flavoring, such as orange, grapefruit, peppermint, nutmeg, etc., with each bringing its different benefits. **Master Formula His and Hers** is a multivitamin formulation made through a 16-stage synergistic suspension isolation to assure that the antagonistic nutrients, like the B-vitamins, don't interfere with the synergistic nutrients, and yet can be put into one tablet.

A third program is for building the immune system. I spent many years developing the **ImmuneTune** formula. Beta carotene always has been respected for its ability to help the body build antibodies, white blood cells, and prevent premature aging and cancer. I also looked at all the difficulties we have when fighting degenerative disease and wanted to incorporate all the ingredients that would help in this area, so I added pantothenic acid, biotin, and coenzyme Q-10. These nutrients always are lacking in people who have degenerative disease. Pycnogynol and essential oils in an herbal base complete the formula.

Pycnogynol is very interesting and needs clarification because of the great controversy regarding its effectiveness. Most of the pycnogynol sold in America is of a very low quality. Again, Americans are more concerned about the cost than the quality, but in reality, the cheaper product costs more in the end. Pure pine pycnogynol has to come from the inner bark or the floam of the tree, which costs $6,800 per kilo. This inner bark is where the active O.P.C. is found, which is the flavonoid responsible for most of the activity. The other three grades of bark have only 6% active O.P.C. or less, depending on how it is processed. It sells for $1,200 per kilo, so the price certainly reflects the quality. The red wine grape pits are even higher in O.P.C. activity; and therefore, by combining the two, the potential results are even greater. The essential oils increase the bio-availability of the nutrients and assist in their delivery to the cells. When combining **ImmuneTune** with **Radex** (which is a powerful free-radical scavenger containing superoxide dismutase), essential oils, and **Super C,** we have an incredible formula for the immune system.

I have been interested not only in the nurturing of the body from the inside but also caring for the body from the outside. I felt it was important to make shampoos and conditioners free of sodium lauryl sulphate, which is one of the leading causes of diminished eyesight in children and allergies in adults. By putting the essential oils in shampoo, I have found that they help oxygenate and cleanse, as well as feed the hair shaft and hair follicle. Lavender, ylang ylang, cedarwood, and rosemary are oils that have been reported to help in the prevention of hair loss and the improvement of hair growth. Sandalwood decreases graying, and rosemary lightens and increases the blond look. Many oils (because of their chelating action) can relax a perm a little early, if used a lot.

After developing allergy symptoms to hand soap from all the chemicals used in my body at the time of my accident, I had a vested interest in making chemical-free soaps. It is an absolute treat to start each day with **Morning Start Bath and Shower Gel**. It is wonderful to nurture the body with life-giving substances, so I have continued to develop more and more products to help protect us and give us a chance against the eroding environment.

When we recognize the incredible attributes in *essential oils* with their *high antioxidant properties, their high antiviral, antibacterial, and anti-infectious properties, their high anti-microbial activity, and their high immune-stimulating power,* one almost would have to conclude that essential oils are truly God's greatest material gift to man.

— RESPONSE PAGE —

I read about Young Living Essential Oils in Lindsey Williams'
new book, *You Can LIVE!* Please send me more information
on essential oils and aromatherapy.

Thank you!

PLEASE PRINT:

Name _____

Address _____

City/State/Zip _____

Telephone (_____) _____

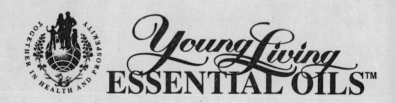

P. O. Box 358
12662 S. Redwood Road
Riverton, UT 84065
(801) 253-2700

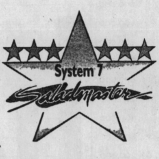

Chapter 9

Cookware For the 21st Century

Saladmaster's Surgical Stainless Cookware

Heart disease! In spite of all our efforts to educate ourselves and adjust our lifestyles, this silent killer continues to sneak up on us. There is a wonderful new publication that I want to recommend (I even have included an order form on the Saladmaster response page at the end of this chapter). It is called *Health Concerns, Twenty-First Century Answers to Today's Health Questions.* It addresses many issues of great concern to us as we reach the close of this century, one of the primary of which is heart disease. The following article is reprinted from the November 1994 edition.

HEART DISEASE STILL #1 KILLER IN U.S.

In 1993, heart disease stole the lives of nearly one million Americans. This is up over 5% of 1983 figures. The present retro-active methods of treating heart disease by drugs and a variety of surgeries is both dangerous and expensive. Another, perhaps more attractive and cost-effective alternative to treating heart ailment is diet and exercise. Treating the cause of heart disease instead of the disease itself is one of the strongest ways to avoid a face-to-face confrontation with America's #1 killer.

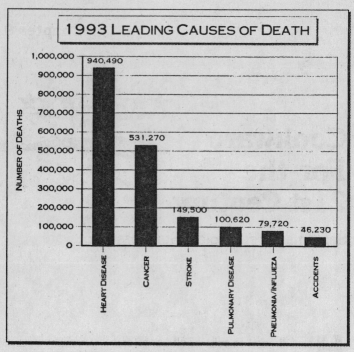

Source: National Center for Health Statistics

What Causes Heart Disease

Psychological stress, cigarette smoking, excessive coffee drinking, and physical inactivity are all factors in the development of coronary heart disease. But perhaps the largest contributor to the nation's largest killer is *diet*. Noted speaker and professor of medicine at Detroit's Wayne State University, Dr. Lawrence Powers said in an interview, "Repeated studies indicate that being overweight, consuming saturated fats and cholesterol are significant factors in dangerously elevating blood cholesterol levels, which produce the coronary heart disease that leads to heart attacks."

Cholesterol & Saturated Fat

A type of fat, called cholesterol, deposits on the walls of arteries, narrowing the passage through which blood flows. This sets the stage for total blockage and the consequential and deadly heart attack, stroke, and high blood pressure. Cholesterol can be found largely in organ meats and egg yolks.

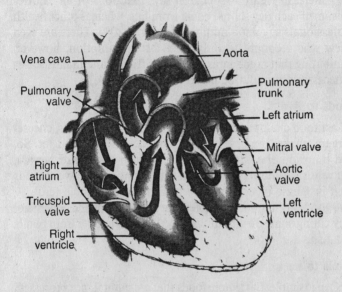

The human heart is an essential machine that, in a lifetime, pumps millions of gallons of blood through arteries the size of wet spaghetti noodles.

Saturated fats, found to increase blood cholesterol levels that promote hardening of the arteries, are found in whole milk, coconut oil, pork fat, and beef fat. Anytime fats and oils are described as "hydrogenated" on food labels, they indeed are saturated and should be avoided.

Unsaturated Fat

Another type of fat, known as unsaturated fat, actually aids in breaking down cholesterol and lowering blood pressure. Foods that contain olive, peanut, and avocado oils, as well as corn, safflower, and sesame oils, are good sources for unsaturated fats.

How Can My Diet Prevent Heart Disease?

Although you won't be able to avoid saturated fats and cholesterol completely, you can reduce your intake of these substances. This, along with increasing your intake of unsaturated fats, will reduce greatly your risk of heart disease. Exactly how much fat we should take in per day is debatable. For example, the American Heart Association says that 30% of all calories consumed each day should come from fats, whereas other health professionals suggest a number of around 20%. There are even a few who recommend only 10% fat consumption, however, eliminating that much fat is not only difficult, and in most cases unnecessary, it could be dangerous.

Foods to Avoid

Fast food chains aren't going to like this. French fries, cheeseburgers, shakes, and pies all are loaded with saturated fat. So, next time you bite into that burger or slurp that shake, **beware**, you've just swallowed enough fat for the entire day. Avoid foods fried in grease or oil, they are high in fat and cholesterol.

A good way to try and counter that saturated fat and cholesterol is by eating some dietary unsaturated fats that come from plants and fish.

Foods to Seek

Keep it simple. Eat simple foods that are natural, not processed, and go for the lowest possible fat content. Eat unlimited fruits and vegetables—all day long! If it grows from the ground and you don't use fats or oil in its preparation, it's good. Eat only a limited amount of fresh nuts (those not processed in oil). Although many fruits, vegetables, and grains have a small amount of fat, it is very difficult to overdose on fats that are still in the fruit, vegetables, or grain.

Except for biscuits, croissants, and dumplings, eat pretty much all the pasta and bread you want. Just be certain that you don't put something with fat or oil on it!! (There are now many fat-free products around.) Discover how convenient bagels, English muffins, and hard rolls are for snacks or for lunch—and they don't crush easily either! They are also a pleasant contrast in texture to fresh stuff.

Limit WHOLE meat to four ounces daily (if you're trying to lose weight) or to the amount you require to hold your weight if you're already at a desirable weight. Hot dogs and sausage are mostly fats, scraps, and salt. Don't eat the skin and trim off any visible fat. Don't fry anything in grease or oil. Use special equipment that allows you to tenderize your food without oil.

Good News!

The GOOD NEWS is you will lose weight, the salt and sugar will take care of themselves, and your heart will be healthier. You'll be likely to spend less money on food. That will put a smile on your face!

DONT'S

No Oils or Fat Added—Some oils are hidden in other products such as mayonnaise or salad dressing. Use FAT-FREE products.

No Junk Food—It's junk food if it has been processed in any other fashion other than drying, crushing, grinding, freezing, or being canned in its own juices or water.

No Fast Food—This stuff is mostly grease.

No Eggs or Dairy products with fat (use only egg substitutes or egg whites, fat-free butter or margarine substitutes, skim or 1% milk, and cheese without fat).

DO'S

Eat All The Fresh Fruits and Vegetables You Want—Just try to take in more than 1500 calories per day of fruits and vegetables (18-20 large bananas, a dozen large apples or oranges, 8-10 white or sweet potatoes, OR two or three quarts of rice cooked below the boiling point to save the important vitamins and minerals!!).

Use Oil-Free, Saladmaster Cookware—This will help keep the nutrients and minerals in the food instead of pouring it all down the drain in the form of discarded boiling water.

Eat All Day—Many small meals help your stomach shrink, but keep it happy. Your blood sugar will stabilize and keep you from screaming in tune with your stomach.

Blow Your Diet—at only one meal a week—and that's **optional!**

Here at Saladmaster, we are happy to recommend this excellent publication. Now, let us introduce a few pertinent *Facts of Life* for your consideration...

- There are mechanics on almost every corner who can grind and reset the valves of your car, but how many doctors do you know who can grind and reset the valves of your heart? It can be done, but it's rather expensive.

- Food should be your medicine...medicine should be your food.
- A great many human ailments can be traced to a faulty diet.
- It *won't* turn out all right, if we don't take control.
- Hospitals are full of people who thought it couldn't happen to them or to their families.
- It's easier to *protect* your health than to *restore* it.
- Luther Burbank: "Violate Nature's Law and the penalty is usually 500 times more than you get."
- The chains of habit are too weak to be felt...*until they are too strong to be broken.*
- King Solomon said: "Timely advice is as lovely as golden apples in a silver basket."
- When you go to the doctor...isn't it true? He takes you off sugar, flour, grease, and salt.
- Some people live long...in spite of what they do; some *because* of it.
- Lasting health comes through proper nutrition. The right foods, plus proper exercise, help you feel and look your best— now and in later years. Isn't it true that we are what we eat?
- Consider this...*Don't gamble with your health!* Why do I say that? If you could not get another car, how carefully would you take care of the one you are driving now? Obviously, that's a rhetorical question. Likewise, you will *never* get another body—this is the one God gave you. So, start taking care of it NOW, by preparing your food *the Saladmaster Way!*

ROBBERS OF GOOD HEALTH

Here are some big enemies to *healthy* and *nutritious* food.

Peeling—In peeling, we eliminate the most nutritious part of our fruits and vegetables. Nutritionists tell us the healthiest part of a potato is within one-eighth inch from the peel. For best health, just scrub your vegetables.

Water—Water leaches out many important minerals from vegetables. Most of the time we pour the water down the drain! Would you pour your fresh coffee down the drain? Instead of boiling your vegetables, tenderize them in a heavy surgical-type stainless steel cooking utensil.

High Heat—This has a tendency to kill the enzymes our bodies require to activate proper food digestion.

Air—Air is disastrous to Vitamin C. Cook in an enclosed, airtight utensil to prevent air from destroying this important nutrient.

Light—Your mother probably taught you about this. Light destroys the color in our home-canned foods. That's why Mom kept those Mason jars in the basement (so light couldn't get to them and turn vegetables white inside the jars).

Grease—This health enemy makes foods seven to eight times harder to digest. Also, the use of grease and added fats to our

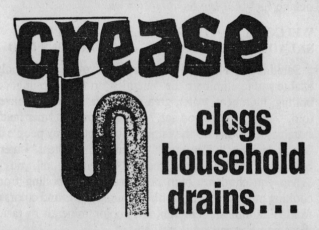

grease clogs household drains...

Think what it could do to your body!

Heart muscles will die if clogged with grease.

Grease can contribute to heart attacks,

obesity and other health problems.

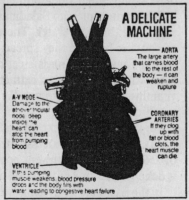

A DELICATE MACHINE

AORTA
The large artery that carries blood to the rest of the body — it can weaken and rupture

A-V NODE
Damage to the atrioventricular node deep inside the heart can stop the heart from pumping blood

CORONARY ARTERIES
If they clog up with fat or blood clots, the heart muscle can die.

VENTRICLE
If this pumping muscle weakens, blood pressure drops and the body fills with water leading to congestive heart failure

Be safe . . . cook the modern, greaseless *Saladmaster* way!!

food prevents our bodies from keeping many of the important
God-given vitamins in our system. For people who are concerned
about living a healthy, happy lifestyle, plan a diet with a lot of
fruits and vegetables, tenderized without boiling. Tenderize in
a life-preserving surgical stainless steel which is designed to cook
foods without grease and water.

Will the motor of your car run without spark plugs? **No!**
Neither can you build your health without minerals and vitamins.
A car knocks and misses on cheap gas—give your body high-
octane fuel. *Eat the Saladmaster way.*

WELCOME TO THE WONDERFUL WORLD OF SALADMASTER HEALTHY & NUTRITIOUS COOKING

Saladmaster Health System provides you with the tools that
enable you to eliminate the "enemies" to food: peeling, coring,
boiling, high heat, water, grease, and air. We always have been
told, "You are what you eat." Years ago, a customer made this
statement: "Don't do the family cooking the way people do the
family laundry." The combination of high heat, water, and
boiling offers the following results, "When you boil, you spoil."
When you eliminate high heat, water, and boiling from the
cooking process, you retain the natural flavors and colors of the
food. Vitamins are represented by color, minerals by taste, and
these complement one another.

When you cook with Saladmaster, you can enjoy food cooked
without grease and water. These are necessary in other forms
of cooking because they spread heat through the food. Saladmaster's unique stainless steel construction evenly distributes
heat, without hot spots, extracting natural juices and leaving
vitamins and minerals intact. We cook foods under low heat and
much quicker.

We know the most expensive food is processed food (canned
food). The canned, processed food is brought to a temperature
of 259°F in order to prevent botulism, and of course, when this
is done, you destroy most of the nutritional benefits of your food.

In the Saladmaster System, we promote use of fresh and frozen
vegetables and meats.

The design and construction offers a 20% savings on the
weekly grocery bill. A demonstration clearly enables a person
to see and understand the savings.

a. A four-pound roast will shrink approximately ⅓ in the oven. Note: if the butcher would cheat the buyer that much, he/she would not continue to trade at that store. You can eliminate that loss by roasting on top of the stove with Saladmaster TP316L Surgical Stainless Steel.

b. In many cases, the doctor will take a patient off sugar, flour, grease, and salt. You can eliminate all four of these in the Saladmaster System.

c. There are five marvelous benefits you can obtain with Salad-master in your home:
   1. More healthful food
   2. Better flavor
   3. Greater convenience
   4. Better appearance
   5. Save money

PHILOSOPHY OF SALADMASTER

Saladmaster cookware is no doubt the best system for *health assurance* that you can have for your kitchen. For the person who believes that their diet has a great deal to do with their health, the Saladmaster cookware will carry a high priority. *Quality health care is not cheap.* All of us know that the body wears out much quicker if we don't feed it properly. So, one of the best *investments* a person can make for their family is to protect their health. A large part of that protection comes from the food you eat...and **how** it is prepared. It is interesting to recall the words of Thomas Edison: "The doctor of the future will give no medicine, but will interest his patients in the care of the human frame, in diet, and in the *cause* and *prevention* of disease."

SALADMASTER ANNOUNCES A NEW LINE: COOKWARE FOR THE 21st CENTURY

The best just keeps getting better! Saladmaster has announced the manufacture and availability of its new "SYSTEM 7" cookware. The unique seven-ply cookware is made using the highest grade and quality of surgical stainless steel available today, TP316L, and is distributed exclusively by Saladmaster. According to Saladmaster President Peter Menke, the recent technological advances made by the steel industry have allowed the company

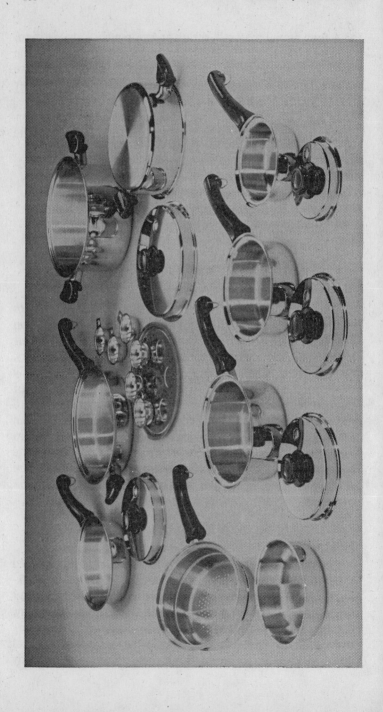

to forge ahead with a superior line of surgical stainless steel cookware. "System 7's unique seven-layer construction features radiant heat-conducting inner layers of aluminum alloys and outer layers of surgical stainless steel for optimum heat distribution," said Menke.

The seven-ply cookware has the added features of over-sized heat guards to prevent fingers from touching hot metal, additional cover height which allows natural moisture to circulate, and a mini-domed lid that creates self-stirring. "This all translates into preserving nutritional values, enhancing food flavors, and saving energy dollars," said Menke. Headquartered in the Dallas area since 1947, Saladmaster is a subsidiary of Regal Ware, Inc. of Wisconsin, and has operations in all 50 states, as well as Canada, Puerto Rico, Australia, Guam, Europe, South Africa, and the Philippines.

Saladmaster System 7 Surgical Stainless Steel cooking utensils are the finest quality products on the market today. Together, they provide a system of waterless and greaseless food preparation which enhances food flavor, while retaining its nutritional value, allowing you to serve better meals, more economically, without diluting natural vitamins and minerals.

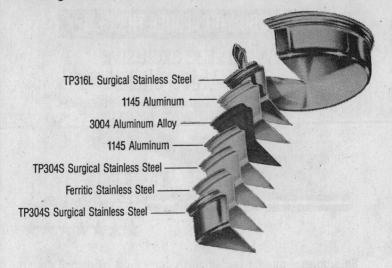

TP316L Surgical Stainless Steel
1145 Aluminum
3004 Aluminum Alloy
1145 Aluminum
TP304S Surgical Stainless Steel
Ferritic Stainless Steel
TP304S Surgical Stainless Steel

The unique multi-layer construction of Saladmaster cookware features radiant heat-conducting inner layers of aluminum alloys and outer layers of surgical stainless steel for optimum heat distribution. This design allows you to cook with minimum heat, saving dollars on your energy bill. The patented VAPO-VALVE™ eliminates guesswork and signals when to turn down the heat. The Vapor Seal Cover creates a semi-vacuum, which shortens cooking time while using a lower temperature setting.

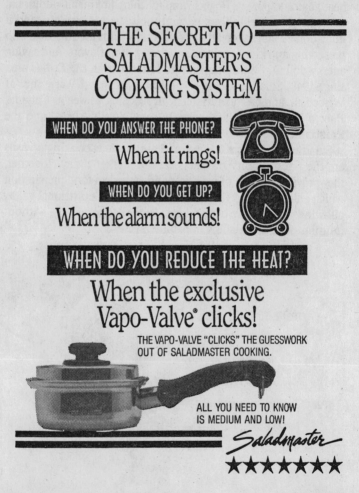

THE SECRET TO SALADMASTER'S COOKING SYSTEM

WHEN DO YOU ANSWER THE PHONE?
When it rings!

WHEN DO YOU GET UP?
When the alarm sounds!

WHEN DO YOU REDUCE THE HEAT?
When the exclusive Vapo-Valve® clicks!

THE VAPO-VALVE "CLICKS" THE GUESSWORK OUT OF SALADMASTER COOKING.

ALL YOU NEED TO KNOW IS MEDIUM AND LOW!

Saladmaster
★★★★★★★

Saladmaster quality is evident in every facet of utensil design. Cool pistol-grip handles, heat-shield knobs, and a dripless pouring edge make serving easier. Clean-up is minimized by rounded corners, which prevent food build-up. High-quality TP316L surgical stainless steel retains its brilliant appearance for many years. Even storage is easier with surgical stainless steel hang-up rings and self-storing lids.

Most important is the Saladmaster guarantee of quality...a lifetime warranty which ensures your cookware will be free from defects in material and workmanship for as long as you own it.

Don't let the *price* of a set of cookware stand in the way of your *good health.* Considering the amount you have invested in your refrigerator, freezer, stove, and other kitchen appliances, doesn't it just make good sense to have cookware that has the capability of capturing and enhancing the nutrition and flavor of your food? These are not just your ordinary "pots and pans." Until you experience the wonderful quality of food prepared in

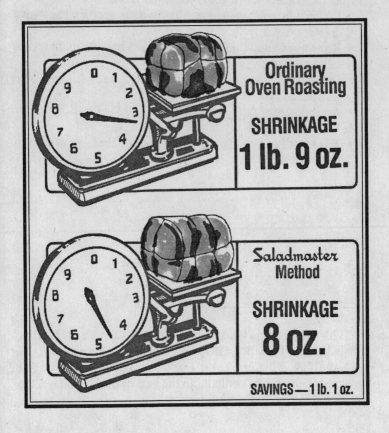

Saladmaster utensils, no words I can use will describe it satisfactorily. I guess the big question is, "Are you getting the picture?" If all you see is "pots and pans," then I have failed...and you have *missed it*. If you see the benefits—more healthful food, convenience, flavor, savings, better appearance of food—then, indeed, you do "get the picture."

Below are some more *Facts of Life*...

- **Priorities**—In the average home, if the TV set went out, it probably would be replaced within 24 hours. Saladmaster utensils, with all their benefits, are much more important to your family than a TV set. Replacements are expensive...you can spend hundreds of dollars and still just have odds and ends. The lifetime warranty extended by Saladmaster is invaluable. The right set of tools for the kitchen is as important as the correct set of tools for a mechanic.
- **Let Saladmaster plug that hole in your grocery bag**—save dollars on yearly food, fuel, etc.
- **Remember,** good things are never cheap, and cheap things are seldom good.
- **Less** food shrinkage, less fuel, no scouring pads, less vegetable loss, no added grease, no replacements.
- **An investment** in Saladmaster will pay for itself.
- **We can purchase** anything except *health*.
- **The health** of your family is worth more than the price of a few pots and pans.

This chapter was written or arranged by Orville E. Martin, Saladmaster, P. O. Box 6183, 6609 Hogue Road, Evansville, IN 47719-0183. Toll-free Phone: 1-800-541-7063. He assumes full responsibiilty for its content. To the best of his knowledge, the material is true and without error.

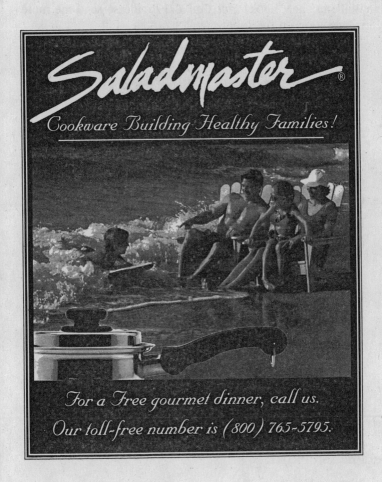

Saladmaster

I read about Saladmaster and *Health Concerns* in Lindsey Williams' new book, *You Can LIVE!* Please send me more information on the following:

☐ Brochures and other information on Saladmaster Stainless Steel Cookware.

☐ Please send me information regarding cookware *not recommended*.

Thank you

PLEASE PRINT:

Name _____

Address _____

City/State/Zip _____

Please make your selection(s) and send to:

AUTHOR	OR	HOME OFFICE
Orville E. Martin		**Saladmaster**
6609 Hogue Road		**912 113th Street**
Evansville, IN 47712		**Arlington, TX 76011**
Toll-Free 1-800-541-7063		**Toll-Free 1-800-765-5795**

☐ Please enter my one-year subscription to *Health Concerns*. Enclosed is my check for $24.00.

☐ Please enter my two-year subscription to *Health Concerns*. Enclosed is my check for $38.40.

Thank you!

PLEASE PRINT:

Name _____

Address _____

City/State/Zip _____

Please make your selection and send with remittance to:

Health Concerns
P. O. Box 202903 • Arlington, TX 76006 • (214) 641-4770

Chapter 10

Plant-Derived Minerals
Mineral Deficiencies—Are You a Victim?

By Patricia Hastings, B.S., N.D.

The rise and fall of past civilizations and their health, by reviewing human history, can be traced to the use or abuse of topsoil. From the earliest civilizations of Egypt, Mesopotamia, Greece, Italy, Sicily and Crete, Western Europe, the Americas, and Asia, as man's soils became depleted and less productive, they would colonize wherever they could find "new land." Since there are no longer "new lands" available to discover and colonize, we presently are faced with the problem of global survival. Man never has learned to be a good steward of his main source of food, *the soil.* If we don't learn from history, we will be plagued with degenerative disease and a shortened life span. In this chapter, I will show you how you can live longer in your generation.

Plants of prehistoric times were rich in minerals; at least 84 to 100 were available. Plants do not have the ability to manufacture minerals; they are limited to absorbing the minerals that are present in the topsoil in which they grow. Plants can make vitamins, amino acids, and essential fatty acids...but not minerals. The mineral content of the world's crops has been decreasing and has been reduced greatly in the last 100 years.

Overgrazing, wind and rain erosion, unwise farming, and continuous cropping all have caused the soils to lack minerals. When early American settlers began to move out across the plains, they would start a small farm, but in two to five years they would pack up the wagon and move farther west. They believed they had "played out the soil," but, in fact, what they did was use up the minerals from the land. A plant is stunted if the soil lacks sufficient minerals. Rich bottom-land farmers could stay in one place because every two to five years there would be a flood, bringing new topsoil and silt to their land, containing 60 or more minerals.

Then in 1908, chemical fertilizers were introduced. The farmer could stay in one place and raise crops over and over again on the same soil. You see, plants only need three minerals to stimulate plant growth and appear lush and beautiful. Have you ever purchased a bag of fertilizer and wondered what those three numbers stood for (10-20-20 or 20-10-10, etc.)? They tell you the ratio of Nitrogen (N), Phosphorus (P), and Potassium (K). That is all plants require—just nitrogen, phosphorus, and potassium—to grow and produce the food we eat. Most farmers never put back more than eight minerals. Even if you eat organically-grown produce, you cannot be guaranteed of healthy mineral content. "Organically grown" just means that no chemical fertilizers or chemical pesticides were used on the crops grown on that soil for the past couple of years. Recently, The Rockland Corporation, in Tulsa, Oklahoma, decided to see what minerals our crops actually contain today. They engaged four leading universities to analyze tomatoes, broccoli, almonds, lettuce, and apples. There were as many as 20 in some cases, but that is a far cry from the 84-100 that once were in our plants.

In the United States, we have taken great pride in our ability to mass-produce food. In fact, we have been called "the breadbasket of the world," because of our abundance of grain. We have shipped grain all over the world to aid in times of shortage and famine. However, the nourishment contained therein is questionable. I believe we are paying a dear price with our health because we have been "strip-mining" our soils, then adding back only three minerals—just enough to make them grow again next season, with even less nutrients than the growing season before. If there once were abundant trace minerals, they now are greatly lacking...or gone entirely, since the plants are unable to generate them. The phrase "over-fed but undernourished" strikes truth, as you will see in this chapter when you discover how vital those trace minerals are to your health and longevity.

Research conducted by the National Science Foundation revealed that animals require at least 45 minerals, 12 essential amino acids, 16 vitamins, and 3 essential fatty acids, and there are federal laws requiring extra minerals in the animal feed. I believe we need 60 or more minerals, but there are no federal laws protecting us—the pets get a better deal. We depend upon our diet from plants first, and secondarily from meats of animals that eat plants, to get our minerals. Unfortunately, there is also a lack of minerals in our meat and dairy products, compared with a few generations ago.

Why are minerals so important to us? They are essential to our physical and mental health. They assist our energy. I have many patients who come in complaining of fatigue. Ninety percent feel better with mineral supplementation. Ninety-six percent of our body is made up of four mineral elements: oxygen, hydrogen, carbon, and nitrogen. Carbon is needed to form vitamins, carbohydrates, fats, lipids, proteins, enzymes, and amino acids. We are two-thirds water (H_2O), therefore, hydrogen plus oxygen is needed. The other 4% of the minerals in our body are comprised of the major minerals (those of which we need 100 mg or more daily) and the trace minerals (those of which our government officials say we need less than 100 mg daily). Many of these trace minerals are lacking in the diet, even if you eat primarily vegetables, fruit, grain, and some meat or fish. There are seven major minerals: calcium, magnesium, potassium, phosphorus, sulfur, sodium, and chlorine. As more nutritional research is conducted, there is more and more evidence that the trace minerals (or lack thereof) have a tremendous impact on our health and longevity. At the end of this chapter, I will let you know how you can get 77 plant-derived colloidal minerals on a daily basis. The body's biochemistry is 95% driven by minerals. Minerals often serve as co-factors or activators in enzymatic systems. Minerals are the basic part of all cells, especially blood, nerves, muscles, bone, teeth, and all soft tissue. If one mineral is missing, physical signs and symptoms can occur, for instance: if soils lack iodine, people living in that area may develop a goiter. In areas in Florida where the soil was deficient in iron (Fe), copper (Cu), and cobalt (Co), 50% or more of the children were found to be anemic.

There is a big difference in the types of minerals:

Elemental or Metallic Minerals are the most difficult to assimilate. We use only 8-12% and after the age of 40 our ability to assimilate this type goes down to approximately 3% to 5%. Examples of this type include clays, rock flours, sea-bed clays, soils, sea-bed minerals, egg shell, oyster shell, calcium carbonate, mineral salt, dolomite, limestone, sea water, Great Salt Lake water, and mineral oxides. This form of mineral is NOT enzymatically alive.

Chelated Minerals—Recognizing the difficulty in assimilation of the elemental or metallic minerals, the natural foods industry came up with a way to increase the bioavailability of the metallic elements. They use a manmade amino acid called EDTA and attach it to the metallic mineral to make a chelated mineral which is 40%-50% bioavailable.

Plant-Derived Colloidal Minerals are a unique class of minerals and are superior to metallic or chelated types because of their small particle size (1/6000th the size of a red blood cell). They are held in suspension, have a negative charge, and are 100% absorbed. They are enzymatically alive if they have been cold-water leached. If they are leached with hot water, acids, or ammonia, they lose their enzymatic principles, even if they were plant-derived colloidal minerals. Plants have taken the elemental or metallic minerals out of the soil through a process known as photosynthesis, digested them for us, and deposited the minerals in their own structure.

Most minerals are not absorbed well. The trace minerals are absorbed very poorly. Some minerals are soluble in water and, therefore, are lost or leached out in the cooking or food preparation process. Many minerals compete with each other when we supplement them or when they are being digested. Large amounts of calcium, for example, can compete with and reduce the absorption of magnesium, manganese, phosphorus, and zinc. Zinc can reduce the absorption of iron, copper, and phosphorus. That is why I recommend and use 77 plant-derived colloidal minerals daily. They are 100% absorbed, and you don't have to worry about absorption competition, as you do with metallic or chelated minerals.

IMPORTANT MINERALS FROM A TO Z

Aluminum (Al) is the third most abundant element in the earth's crust, after oxygen and silicon. It is very common in plants and is found in most food we eat. There have been many studies connecting disease with metallic aluminum, even a possible connection with Alzheimer's disease. For that very reason, over the last 20 years I have avoided aluminum cookware and products with metallic aluminum. But I eat *lettuce, potatoes, wheat,* and *tomatoes* that contain plant-derived colloidal aluminum on a daily basis. Don't feel bad if you have been confused about products with plant-derived colloidal aluminum in them. Even leading nutritional doctors and leaders of countries such as Finland did not know the difference. Finland is now in the process of changing their federal law because it was unlawful to consume more than 2 mg of aluminum daily. They made no distinction between metallic aluminum and plant-derived colloidal aluminum. When they became aware that the plant-derived colloidal form was not harmful, and that their law would make it illegal to eat more than just a sliver of a banana, they took steps to change it.

Here are some results from the *ATL Agronomy Handbook,* under the section "Plant Analysis Guide Nutrient Sufficiency Ranges." PPM and Mg/L (parts per million and milligrams per liter) are considered equal since there are 994,000 mg in one liter.

Plant Food	Aluminum in PPM	Plant Food	Aluminum in PPM
Asparagus	90	Oil Palm	98
Bananas	97	Peas	45
Beans	165	Peanuts	75
Brussels Sprouts	65	Peppers	75
Celery	190	Pineapple	100
Coffee	97	Potatoes	100
Corn (at tasseling)	140	Root Crops	140
Cucumbers	90	Small Grains	135
Head Crops (lett.)	90	Soybeans	75
Leaf Crops	50	Tomatoes	90
Melons	65	Wheat	140
Mint	140		

Arsenic (As) is found in many foods, for instance apples and tomatoes. Studies have shown it may prevent TMJ, carpel tunnel syndrome, and certain tendon problems. Once again, metallic arsenic can kill you, but plant-derived colloidal arsenic is not harmful and may be beneficial in trace amounts.

Bismuth (Bi) is nontoxic in normal amounts. It is the active ingredient in Pepto-Bismol.

Boron (B) helps maintain calcium balance, prevents osteoporosis, and keeps bones healthy. It is required to maintain levels of Vitamin D and certain hormones, including testosterone and estrogen. I encourage all my patients, especially menopausal and postmenopausal women, to take extra boron daily. For decades, boric acid has been used topically as an eyewah and antiseptic for the skin. It also plays a role in preventing hypertension and arthritis due to balancing calcium by regulating the parathyroid.

Cadmium (Cd) in its metallic form is toxic, but is nontoxic in its plant-derived form.

Calcium (Ca) is one of the most difficult minerals to absorb, which is why I recommend the plant-derived colloidal form, which is 100% assimilated. The major and minor symptoms of a calcium deficiency are many: osteoporosis, tooth decay, insomnia, muscle aches and cramps, muscle twitching, tetany, PMS, high blood pressure, arthritis, bone spurs, rickets, failure to thrive, poor growth, osteomalacia, neuromuscular disorders, nervousness, heart palpitations, numbness of the limbs, irritability, brittle fingernails, depressions, delusions, eczema, hyperactivity, and decreased cognitive reasoning.

Carbon (C) is needed to produce vitamins, enzymes, amino acids, carbohydrates, and fats.

Cerium (Ce) has antiseptic properties. It has been used as a topical disinfectant and on severe burns.

Cesium (Cs) as cesium chloride currently is being used to produce an alkaline environment in the cancer cell in some cancer therapies.

Chlorine (Cl) activates enzyme systems and is an important component of HCL (our stomach acid). It also functions as an electrolyte in the form of chloride and works with sodium and water to distribute the body fluids. It is helpful in allowing the liver to clear waste products, and it maintains the body's acid-base balance.

Chromium (Cr) along with vanadium (Va) helps in diabetes and hypoglycemia by regulating blood glucose levels. If lacking, it has been connected to anxiety, depression, biopolar disorder, poor growth, attention deficit disorder (ADD), hyperactivity, infertility, elevated cholesterol and triglycerides, and a shortened lifespan.

Cobalt (Co) is the core of Vitamin B12 (cobalamine). Cobalt is a co-factor and is necessary in the production of thyroid hormones.

Copper (Cu) has a key function as an enzyme co-factor. It is important in the formation of hemoglobin, our oxygen-carrying molecule. It is part of an energy-releasing process—the cytochrome system for cellular respiration, involved in energy production. Copper supports the healing process, aids in bone formation, works with Vitamin C to form collagen, which is a supportive matrix in muscle, bone, and connective tissue. It contributes to the integrity of the myelin sheath covering nerves. It helps to convert T3 to T4 (thyroid hormones). If copper is deficient, the thyroid shows decreased function, including fatigue, weight gain, and low basal body temperature and metabolic rate. Copper protects us from aortic and cerebral aneurysms. It aids in the conversion of tyrosine to the pigment melanin which gives hair and skin their color. I have seen many patients' hair restore from white or gray to its original color with the use of the plant-derived colloidal minerals that contain colloidal copper. Gray hair will regain its color if it was due to lack of minerals, especially copper.

Dysprosium (Dy) is found in the bones.

Erbium (Er) is found in bones.

Europium (Eu) had doubled the normal life expectancy in laboratory animals.

Fluorine (Fl) has a key function in strengthening the structure of bones and teeth. It is nontoxic in its plant-derived colloidal form.

Gadolinium (Gd) is found in the liver and bones.

Gallium (Ga) is involved in enzymatic activity in the brains of humans. In both children and lab animals, studies have shown a decrease in cancer rates of the brain when their mothers were supplied gallium while pregnant.

Holmium (Ho) is found in the bones.

Hydrogen (H) is involved in the acid-balance regulation in the body, as well as in the regulation of intracellular and extracellular body fluids. We are two-thirds water (H_2O). It also has a key function in the tissues of the body.

Iodine (I) is essential in the synthesis of the thyroid hormones, especially thyroxine which is 65% iodine. The thyroid hormones are responsible for the body's use of energy, the basal metabolic rate (BMR). Our BMR affects almost all of our body functions, our production of energy as ATP, and our general metabolism. If iodine is lacking, a person may develop a goiter, hyperthyroidism, sluggishness, fatigue, difficulty in concentration, decreased libido (sex drive), muscle aches and pains, dry hair or hair loss, weight gain, low basal body temperature and low metabolic rate, brittle nails, constipation, puffiness in the face, and feeling cold. A deficiency of iodine may increase the risk of breast cancer. Iodine in its colloidal form is beneficial, but in its free form, even two grains would kill you.

Iron (Fe) has a key function in hemoglobin which is an oxygen carrier. If lacking in the diet, it can lead to iron-deficiency anemia (hypochromic microcytic anemia), anorexia, constipation, depression, fatigue, sore tongue, irritability, confusion, brittle fingernails, heart palpitations, dizziness, indigestion, headaches, and fragile bones. Copper deficiency usually accompanies iron-deficiency anemia.

Lanthanum (La) has been shown to double life expectancy in lab species.

Lead (Pb) is toxic in the metallic form, but is nontoxic in its plant-derived colloidal form.

Lithium (Li) generates a sweeter outlook toward life and it strengthens the immune system. It is used in the treatment of depression, bipolar manic depression, and alcoholism. Lithium is involved in several hundred enzymatic reactions, many of which contribute to energy production and cardiac function.

Lutetium (Lu) is found in soft tissue and bones.

Magnesium (Mg) is important in bone structure, muscle control, and is an antispasmodic. It is a co-enzyme activator of Vitamin B1 in the oxidation of carbohydrates and is important in the cell's production of energy. It is a metabolic electrolyte. Magnesium, along with potassium supplementation can reduce fatigue. The many enzyme systems that require magnesium as a co-factor help restore normal energy levels. Caffeine, sugar, stress, alcohol, and diuretic drugs can lead to magnesium loss. When magnesium is deficient, the following major and minor symptoms may occur: muscle weakness, bronchial restriction in asthma, neuromuscular problems, tetany, ECG changes, coronary artery spasms, heart attacks, high blood pressure, calcification of the small arteries and soft tissue, asthma, depression, menstrual cramps, PMS, menstrual migraines, vertigo, tremors, failure to thrive, anorexia, kidney stones, irritability, tingling, muscle twitching, tachycardia (rapid heart beat). Magnesium may aid in the prevention of kidney stones, especially calcium oxalate stones, by increasing the solubility of calcium in urine.

Manganese (Mn) is involved in glucose metabolism, protein metabolism, and bone formation. It activates a number of enzymes necessary for the body to use Vitamins B1, biotin, choline, and Vitamin C. It is involved with the production of energy, SOD, the synthesis of L-dopamine. If a deficiency occurs, one might experience fatigue, poor memory, dizziness, irritability, nervousness, tendon disorders, TMJ, strange ear noises, convulsions and seizures, paralysis, carpel tunnel syndrome, infertility, asthma, joint and bone cartilage problems, and deafness.

Mercury (Hg) as a plant-derived colloidal form can protect us from selenium poisoning, as does selenium protect us from mercury poisoning.

Molybdenum (Mo) is an enzyme co-factor that activates many enzyme systems. It now is considered an essential trace mineral. It recently was discovered that the soil in certain areas of China was responsible for the highest known incidence of esophageal carcinoma in over many generations. The soil was greatly deficient in molybdenum. Molybdenum can reduce or counteract the action of nitrosamine, which is a known cancer-causing chemical. Molybdenum has antioxidant properties and may prevent anemia by mobilizing stored iron from the liver.

Neodymium (Nd) has been shown to double normal life expectancy in laboratory species.

Nickel (Ni) may involve hormone, lipid, and membrane metabolism. If deficiency occurs, it may delay puberty, affect normal growth, cause rough, dry hair and dermatitis, anemia, liver disorders, and cause poor zinc absorption.

Nitrogen (N) is a structural ingredient in protein, DNA, and

RNA. If it is lacking, it leads to poor growth, edema, kwashior-
kor disease, infertility, and a decreased immune system.

Oxygen (O) has an essential role in cellular and tissue respiration, which produces energy. Without oxygen, our life ends
quickly. The earth's atmosphere once had 50% oxygen, but now
it only has about 19%, according to U.S. geologists. Oxygen also
is a major component in the water in our bodies.

Phosphorus (P) is in all foods. Its key role is in our bones
and teeth. The following symptoms may occur if there is a
deficiency of phosphorus: paresthesia (a shooting pain down the
back of the legs), numbness, irritability, fatigue, anxiety, bone
pain, weakness, tremulousness, or weight loss.

Potassium (K) is essential for our physical and mental well
being. When it is lacking or deficient, mental apathy sets in, as
well as muscle weakness, irregular heart beats, and cardiac
failure. It maintains the alkali balance in our blood plasm and
transmits electrical impulses along the neuromuscular path which
influences the heart.

Praseodymium (Pr) has been shown to double the normal life
expectancy in laboratory species.

Rubidium (Rb) has a possible tranquilizing effect on the body;
it can replace the electrolyte function of potassium. It is used
in the treatment of epilepsy and nervous disorders.

Samarium (Sm) has been shown to double the normal life
expectancy in lab species.

Selenium (Se) was considered a nonessential toxic mineral just
20 years ago. Now, it is considered an essential trace mineral.
It has a key function as an enzyme co-factor, an antioxidant,
and aids in detoxification. Major and minor deficiency symptoms
include an increase in cancer risk, heart attack, cataracts, kidney
disease, cystic fibrosis, sterility in men, liver cirrhosis, high blood
pressure, muscular dystrophy, growth retardation, eczema,
psoriasis, cervical dysplasia, alcoholism, infections, rheumatoid
arthritis, decreased immunity, and myocardial fibrosis. Increased
cancer rates have been shown to be associated with low soil levels
of selenium. Keshan disease is a heart disease in children. It leads
to an enlarged heart and congestive heart failure. The disease
was discovered in Keshan, China, where there were low levels
of selenium in the soil. Selenium may prevent our number-one
and number-two killer diseases: cardiovascular disease and

cancer.

Silicon (Si) aids in the development of growing bones, teeth, collagen, and connective tissue. It may help lower cholesterol. If deficient, symptoms may include dry brittle hair, poor skin quality, brittle finger and toe nails, calcium utilization will be decreased, arterial disease, lower stamina, atherosclerosis, and heart disease.

Silver (Ag) has been used for thousands of years by some cultures and is gaining popularity today as an immune system enhancer and systemic disinfectant. Other forms of silver can produce side effects, but the plant-derived colloidal form does not. In my practice, it has helped in the healing process, topically and internally for lesions, shown great reduction of inflammation, especially in enlarged prostates, bladder irritation, shingles, and a number of other infections. It is nontoxic in normal rates of consumption and is an antibacterial, antifungal, antiviral mineral. In *Science Digest,* March 1978, the article "Silver: Our Mightiest Germ Fighter" reported silver to be an antibiotic that can kill over 650 disease-causing invaders.

Sodium (Na) maintains normal water balance of cellular fluids, normalizes osmotic pressure in the blood plasma, maintains the acid-base balance of the body. Its key function is as an extracellular electrolyte. Sodium deficiency symptoms include: weight loss, seizures, depression, bouts of crying, confusion, abdominal cramps, anorexia, fatigue, dizziness, headaches, increased infection, memory loss, loss of taste, muscle weakness, nausea, vomiting, and flatulence.

Strontium (Sr) is found in bones, and if deficient, it can lead to osteoporosis and arthritis, increased tooth decay, poor calcification of bones and teeth. It has a key function in bone strength and integrity. Nonradioactive strontium is beneficial to our bones and teeth. It is nontoxic and occurs naturally in food.

Sulfur (S) has a key function in enzyme reactions and protein synthesis. It helps form collagen, the protein found in connective tissue. It is necessary for cellular respiration and maintains healthy skin, nails, and hair. It is involved in the structure of carbohydrates, most protein, and some hormones, such as insulin and adrenal corticol hormone. If sulfur is deficient, a variety of symptoms may develop, such as collagen disease, degenerative arthritis, tendinitis, degeneration of the cartilage and of ligaments. Sickle cell anemia and lupus (SLE) also have been linked to a sulfur deficiency.

Terbium (Tb) is found in the bones.

Thulium (Tm) has been shown to enhance growth in normal cells and double the life expectancy in laboratory species.

Tin (Sn) may play a role in protein structure, oxidation, and reduction reactions. It has been shown to prevent hair loss and hearing loss. It also plays a role in proper growth. Tin does not work in isolation, but instead with other trace minerals such as copper and iron.

Vanadium (Va) has shown the ability, along with chromium, to regulate blood glucose levels in diabetics and hypoglycemics. It also plays a key role in lipid metabolism. If deficient, it can lead to failure to thrive, poor growth, infant mortality, obesity, cardiovascular disease, increased cholesterol, increased tryglycerides, and infertility.

Yttrium (Y) has shown that it aids normal cell growth and doubles the life expectancy of laboratory species.

Zinc (Zn) aids immune function and promotes the healing of wounds and ulcers. Deficiency states can lead to birth defects (e.g., spina bifida, cleft lip and palate, clubbed limbs, webbed toes and fingers called syndactyl), anemia, hair loss, brittle nails, acne, eczema, boils, psoriasis, sore throats, colds, gastric ulcers, hiatal hernia, weight loss, diarrhea, memory loss, white spots on the nails, malabsorption, poor growth, severe body odor, depression, benign prostatic hypertrophy, anorexia, fatigue, loss of taste, hypercholesterolemia, infertility, impotence, sterility, high blood pressure, alcoholism, and muscle weakness.

There is a crisis with our soils lacking the abundance of minerals they once contained. After reading the section "Important Minerals from A to Zinc," I believe you see how important the full spectrum of minerals is to our health and longevity. The answer is to *supplement.* But how can you find some of these rare earth trace minerals? If you did find them, it would cost too much to take each one separately. How would you know the right proportions of each one, and as I pointed out, it needs to be in the plant-derived colloidal form.

My prayers were answered when I found out about a prehistoric plant deposit of humic shale in Emery County, Utah. It was entombed under high pressure and did not get enough moisture to petrify, nor was it carbonized in order to turn to coal. It was discovered in 1926. By 1930, methods of extracting the minerals from the humus with a cold-water leaching process revealed it contained over 60 colloidal minerals made from plants, not ground up soil or rocks. It was introduced as "Body Toddy" in 1984 by The Rockland Corporation. The name was changed to "Mineral Toddy," and subsequently, the name was sold. Presently, The Rockland Corporation sells the pure, unadulterated minerals under the name of "Body Booster™." The water has been eliminated by low-temperature evaporation, to make a capsule-form of the 77 Plant-Derived Colloidal Minerals. It sells under the Liquid Assets division of The Rockland Corporation. Rockland has a 1,000-acre mining lease, which contains approximately 32 million metric tons of humic shale, which is enough to produce 950 billion gallons of the liquid Body Booster™ minerals. I have been to the mines in Emery County and realize the impact these minerals can have on our health and longevity. Emery County has the only known source of this type of "Mother Nature-produced" minerals. The Rockland Corporation maintains extremely high standards in its mining, leaching process, and bottling techniques.

We are extremely excited about the Body Booster™ capsules because of their convenience. No refrigeration, no measuring or spilling, no unpleasant taste; my granddaughters, April and Kim, thought the liquid form tasted "disgusting" (their words). Easy long-term storage (forever), use for travel, and shipping all make the Body Booster™ capsules the way to supply the missing minerals the body needs and on which it depends for optimal health. Order yours today using the convenient response page at the end of this chapter. Good health and God bless you!

Patricia Hastings, B.S., N.D.

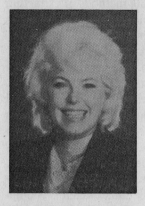

Dr. Patricia Hastings has been involved in wholistic health for more than 40 years. She has a Bachelors of Science (B.S.), with human biology as her major and chemistry her minor. Her master herbalist degree (M.H.) was obtained from the Emerson College of Herbology. Her thesis for her Master's degree in Nutrition was written on Diabetes. Dr. Hastings earned her Naturopathic Doctor degree from Bastyr University of Naturopathic Medicine in Seattle in 1983 and currently serves on the Board of Trustees. She served on the Center for Health Statistics Advisory Committee for the Washington State Department of Health. She has been President of the Washington Association of Naturopathic Physicians for four years. Dr. Hastings is director of the Northwest Wholistic Health Center, which she founded in 1983, in Olympia, Washington. She is a family practice physician, dealing with acute and chronic illness through nutritional and botanical therapies. For an appointment, call (360) 438-2882. She is the National Marketing Field Director for the Liquid Assets Division of The Rockland Corporation. Her toll-free number for Liquid Assets products is 1-800-680-6742, or call The Rockland Corporation at 1-800-492-4995.

BODY BOOSTER™ CAPS

Body Booster™ is not only the most famous plant-derived liquid mineral, it is also the purest, most concentrated, comprehensive, and result-producing plant mineral in the world. The Rockland Corporation introduced Body Booster™ to the multi-level industry under the name Body Toddy in 1984. The Body Toddy name subsequently was changed to Mineral Toddy. The Mineral Toddy name was sold, however, the unaltered mineral product is still available from Rockland as Body Booster™.

Each quart of Body Booster™ contains approximately 38,000 milligrams of a natural assortment of 77 minerals, which are leached —with cool, contaminant-free water—from a prehistoric plant material known as Humic Shale. This shale is extracted from The Rockland Mine in Emery County, Utah.

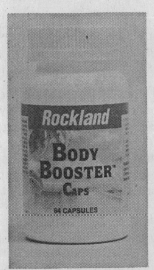

Due to the weight and space requirements of liquids, Body Booster™ has been burdensome to its loyal users. This also created a freight and handling problem. The company now has found a way to circumvent these obstacles. A low-temperature drying method was developed to remove the water from Body Booster™. The remaining powder is equal to the solids of the preceding liquid and contains a natural assortment of 77 plant-derived colloidal minerals. This powdered mineral, which never is subjected to temperatures above 84°F during the drying process, is now available from Liquid Assets in 600 milligram capsules. **It is known as Body Booster™ Caps.** Each capsule is equivalent to ½ ounce of the original Body Booster™. Two capsules with a glass of water or juice is the identical dosage as one liquid ounce of Body Booster™ or Rockland's former Body Toddy.

Each Body Booster™ capsule contains 600 milligrams of the following 77 plant-derived minerals:

Calcium	Cadmium	Holmium	Nitrogen	Tantalum
Chlorine	Carbon	Hydrogen	Osmium	Tellurium
Magnesium	Cerium	Indium	Oxygen	Terbium
Phosphorus	Cesium	Iodine	Palladium	Thallium
Potassium	Chromium	Iridium	Platinum	Thorium
Sodium	Cobalt	Iron	Praseodymium	Thulium
Sulfur	Copper	Lanthanum	Rhenium	Tin
Antimony	Dysprosium	Lead	Rhodium	Titanium
Arsenic	Erbium	Lithium	Rubidium	Tungsten
Aluminum	Europium	Lutetium	Ruthenium	Vanadium
Hydroxide	Fluorine	Manganese	Samarium	Ytterbium
Barium	Gadolinium	Mercury	Scandium	Yttrium
Beryllium	Gallium	Molybdenum	Selenium	Zinc
Bismuth	Germanium	Neodymium	Silicon	Zirconium
Boron	Gold	Nickel	Silver	
Bromine	Hafnium	Niobium	Strontium	

— RESPONSE PAGE —

Dear Dr. Hastings:

I read about Body Booster™ Caps in Lindsey Williams' new book, *You Can LIVE!*

☐ I want to try Body Booster™ Caps. Please send me the initial order of 4 bottles (64 caps per bottle). Enclosed is my check in the amount of $110.00, which includes shipping.

☐ I am interested in other products from Liquid Assets/Rockland Corporation. Please send me a descriptive catalog or brochure, with ordering information.

Thank you!

PLEASE PRINT UPS SHIPPING ADDRESS (No P.O. boxes):

Name _____

Street Address _____

City/State/Zip _____

Telephone (_____) _____

Please make your selection(s) and send to:

Dr. Patricia Hastings
4324 Martin Way
Olympia, WA 98516
TOLL-FREE Order Number 1-800-680-6742

Chapter 11

H₂O

America's Drinking Water Crisis

What You *Don't* Know About It Could Kill You!

By Lyle Loughry & Jonathon Miller
UltraSource, Inc.

This chapter is submitted as a basic primer on the subject of water, and water for personal use in particular.

THE PHENOMENON WE CALL WATER

The origin of water is as open to speculation as the origin of the earth itself. What we know for certain is that it exists *today*, covering approximately three-fourths of the earth's surface—some 326 million cubic feet of it—and that 97% of it is in the oceans. *The remaining 3% is available to us as "fresh water."* Unfortunately, three-fourths of that 3% is frozen in glaciers and ice caps. The remaining one-fourth of the 3% is found underground, in lakes, rivers, and in the atmosphere.

Our earth possesses a *fixed* supply of water. There never will be more of it than there is now. The *hydrologic cycle* is nature's way of purifying the earth's water. The process used is that of evaporation (turning to vapor) and precipitation (condensing moisture from a vaporous state back into rain, snow, etc.). Through this process, used quantities of water always will return to the earth. In short, water is reusable and recyclable. In fact, every glass of water you drink contains water molecules that have been around since the earth began—cleansed repeatedly through nature's enormous distillation system.

Almost every civilization was born and cradled on the banks of the earth's great rivers. Even so, to some extent we all take water for granted. This was not always the case. Water, along with fresh air, was the orthodox medical treatment of ancient Greece, Rome, and Egypt. In practically all ancient religions, pure water was used for the purification of the body and was referred to as "holy," because it was known to heal. The quality of their drinking water was the most important factor in the Greek way of life, and it is said that the Greeks reached a standard of clear thinking and physical perfection that never has been surpassed.

Water is as essential to life as the air we breathe. While the human body will survive up to two months without solid food, it cannot live much longer than five days without water. All living organisms—plant and animal, which includes humans—consist mostly of water. When we are born, our bodies are about 97% water. When we reach adulthood, our bodies are about 70% water, although even then our blood composition remains approximately 92% water.

The water within us is vital to our life-sustaining function: breathing, circulation, digestion, glandular activities, heat dissipation, and secretion. Through the processes of perspiration and elimination alone, the body loses 3-8 pints daily. In order to maintain health, this water must be replaced each day. In addition to the liquid in the food we ingest and the beverages we drink, *we also need 3 to 4 pints of purified water each day.*

Plants live on the food they make themselves from water, sunlight, carbon dioxide, and inorganic minerals. The absorption and release of carbon dioxide by the world's water is used to control the balance of gasses in our atmosphere. Truly, water is a special blessing and benefit, without which we could not survive.

Next to oxygen, water is the substance we need most, but suspect least. However, recent public opinion polls reveal an alarming increase in the concern shown over the widespread pollution of the earth's water supplies.

THE PROBLEM WITH OUR DRINKING WATER SUPPLIES

The social, industrial, and technological advances we all enjoy have created an ever-increasing demand on our fresh water supplies. This, in turn, has necessitated the *re-use of our water before it has time to enter the "Hydrologic Cycle" for cleansing.* Remember what we said earlier about our water supply being constant? We have to work with what we have! As a result, we have had to *substitute manmade processes for nature's purification process.* Therein lies a very big problem!

Without attempting to trace the deterioration in quality of the earth's water supply through the centuries, we will look more specifically at the events of the 20th century. Virtually the world over, sanitation procedures are necessary to rid public drinking supplies of pollutants—from the simplest "natural" pollutants, i.e., mineral deposits, bacteria, and viruses, to "organic" contaminants, i.e., detergents, fertilizers, pesticides, and gasoline, in addition to an ever-increasing number of "inorganic" pollutants, i.e., acids, mining wastes, lead, mercury, and toxic waste spills. Add to these, radioactive substances and thermal pollution, and you begin to see the enormity of the problem we face, and why there is a *recognized water crisis* in much of our world (even more so in developed, industrialized countries).

A 1976 EPA study listed 32,254 disposal sites with potentially hazardous wastes leaking into the underground water supply, poisoning the drinking water. According to another EPA study, municipal sewers discharge *40 billion gallons,* industry *125 billion gallons,* and agriculture *50 billion gallons* of waste DAILY into our water sources. *Each year 1,700 billion gallons of waste liquids are placed into the ground, of which 800 billion gallons are human waste!*

The list of towns, cities, and farms that suffer from contaminants is endless!

THE EXTENT OF THE PROBLEM

According to a 1977 U.S. Government report, over 400 organic chemicals alone have been discovered in America's drinking water. Such organic chemicals—often by-products of dead leaves, humus, trash, and animal wastes—occur naturally in water systems, or run off the land into them, or enter them as sewage.

Over 2,000,000 synthetic organics are known to exist, and 25,000 are added each year. Unknown are their potentially devastating synergistic effects.

The most insidious chemicals and pollutants found in our drinking water are colorless, odorless, and tasteless. *Just because water looks good, smells good, and tastes good does not mean that it is good for you!*

Inorganic solutes (dissolved substances) are a category of water contaminants comprised of the following minerals: barium, beryllium, cadmium, chromium, cobalt, copper, lead, magnesium, manganese, mercury, molybdenum, nickel, potassium, silver, sodium, tin, vanadium, and zinc. While many of these minerals can be healthful in small amounts, large toxic levels of many of them are found in much of America's water supplies, most notably lead, *a cumulative poison easily concentrated in the body,* and mercury. According to the United States Environmental Protection Agency (EPA), "...as many as one in four Americans may be drinking water which contains levels of lead dangerous enough to cause various health problems, such as miscarriages, birth defects, mental and physical retardation in young children, even the lowering of children's intelligence quotient (IQ)."

Approximately 80% of the mercury used around the world is discharged into the environment. It is extremely toxic, and its effects may not appear for months or years after initial absorption.

The Council on Environmental Quality reports that a typical moderate-sized city annually discharges 100,000 to 250,000 pounds of lead; 6,000 to 30,000 pounds of mercury; 15,000 to 30,000 pounds of chromium; 85,000 to 90,000 pounds of copper; 140,000 to 300,000 pounds of zinc; and over 10,000 pounds of nickel—not to mention human waste!

The relatively clean water that flows out of Canada and through America's northern border states picks up chemical run-offs, industrial spills, municipal discharges, toxic dumping, etc., in state after state as it journeys southward to the Gulf of Mexico and beyond. One only can cringe at the increasingly deplorable condition of this once-pristine commodity as it heads south.

According to EPA figures released in *Prevention Magazine,* "...63% of rural residences drink contaminated water."

"Contemporary treatment plants are not equipped to effectively remove most metals and trace elements, synthetic chemicals and radionuclides from our water supplies, and *50% of the U.S. population use water that, in part, is made up of recently discharged wastewater*" [emphasis added] (*The State of Drinking Water in America,* Dunne, 1977).

THE SOLUTION TO THE PROBLEM?

Efforts to treat water and remove pollutants during this century have employed procedures ranging from *aeration* (the charging or treating of water with air), to *sedimentation* (the holding of water to allow for the sediment suspended in the water to accumulate), to *chlorination* (the treatment of water with the poisonous chemical gas, chlorine, first introduced in 1908), to *filtration* (the introduction of a substance, such as cloth, paper, porous porcelain, charcoal, or sand, through which the water is passed to remove suspended impurities, or to recover solids).

By far, *chlorination* has been the most popular single treatment, and it is used almost universally as the treatment of choice to remove bacteria from water supplies. *Bacteria can kill people,* so this problem was—and still is—the foremost concern of those who manage municipal water supplies, large and small.

These treatments seemed to be effective early in this century, but in the last 30 years have been determined by many leading researchers to be inadequate. At one time, the claim that America's public water supplies were "the best in the world" went unchallenged; today, the taste, odor, chemicals, and bacteria count of what flows out of the tap literally can make you sick—*or kill you!*

It is safe to conclude that water supples in other countries, especially those which have experienced industrial expansion in the 20th century, have been overwhelmed similarly. Evidence reveals that in most instances they are in even worse condition.

THE PROBLEM WITH THE SOLUTION

Water treatment hasn't changed much since 1908 when chlorine first was introduced. What has changed is our awareness of the hidden dangers of the chemical itself. Even so, chlorine still is used extensively to kill bacteria in municipal water supplies. Almost from the beginning, chlorine has had its critics. Concerned biologists and environmentalists have been on the trail of carcinogens in disinfected drinking water for a long time, but only in the past 20 years have such investigations gained national attention.

Most medical researchers were led to believe that chlorine was safe, but they now have learned that, while in the process of preventing epidemics of typhoid, cholera, and dysentery, we have created others. According to Joseph M. Price, M.D., author and noted chlorine researcher, "Chlorine has become the greatest crippler and killer of modern times, and the cause of an unprecedented disease epidemic, which includes cancer, heart attacks, senility, sexual impotency, and strokes."

The general public, and most water treatment officials, still believe chlorination remains the solution to making water safe. **NOT SO!** According to The National Academy of Sciences, "Chlorine interacts with naturally-found humus and humic acid (both products of decaying plant matter) to form THM's (trihalomethanes). The most common of the THM's is chloroform, which can cause liver and kidney damage, central nervous system depression, and is a human carcinogen."

Francis T. Mayo, Director, Municipal Environment Research Laboratory, declares: "Trihalomethanes in general, and chloroform, a known carcinogen in particular, are found in drinking water as a *direct consequence of the practice of chlorination*, a long-established health practice for the disinfection of drinking water" [emphasis added].

According to Lance Wallace, EPA scientist, "Showering is suspected as the primary cause of elevated levels of chloroform in nearly every home in America, because of the chlorine in the water."

In 1974, the EPA and a Dutch scientist each reported the presence of chlorine-related carcinogens in treated drinking water. The same year, the Environmental Defense Fund, a nonprofit group, released findings of a year-long study showing that people in southern Louisiana who derived drinking water from the Mississippi River had *10% to 20% more fatal cancer* in organs of the gastrointestinal and urinary tracts than people living in other parts of the state who drank water from other sources.

In 1975, the EPA discovered chloroform and other carcinogens in measurable amounts in the drinking water systems of 80 communities in the nation, including the District of Columbia,

Baltimore, Philadelphia, Cincinnati, Miami, and Seattle.

In 1976, the Ohio State University's Comprehensive Cancer Center conducted a nationwide 200-county study of cancer mortality and chlorinated water supplies. They found increased rates of fatal cancer of the bladder and large intestines in older persons, particularly those over 60.

According to biological chemist Dr. Herbert Schwartz, Cumberland County College, "Chlorine has so many dangers it should be banned. Putting chlorine into the water supply is like starting a time bomb. Cancer, premature senility—both mental and physical—are conditions attributable to chlorine-treated water supplies. It makes us grow old before our time by producing symptoms of aging, such as hardening of the arteries. *When you drink chlorinated water, you should expect a premature end of cell-life!*" [emphasis added].

According to a recent study of the U.S. Council of Environmental Quality, "Cancer risk among people drinking chlorinated water is 93% higher than among those whose water does not contain chlorine."

In July 1992, researchers at the Harvard University School of Public Health and the Medical College of Wisconsin, in studies published in *The American Journal of Public Health,* revealed that: "Chlorine used in municipal water supplies to kill germs may create chemical compounds that make people more susceptible to cancers of the bladder and rectum."

Recently, after conducting a 16-month water quality control study for the U.S. EPA, Dr. John Cristman, Director of Research, Loyola University, concluded, *"Home water treatment systems may be the only feasible way of ensuring that water is fit to drink"* [emphasis added].

An article appearing in the September 26, 1993, *New York Times Magazine* revealed: "Much of America's tap water is inadequately monitored, and possibly unsafe." The article mentioned in particular the April, 1993, cryptosporidiosis outbreak (an illness caused by a water-borne parasite) that sickened 400,000 residents in Milwaukee, Wisconsin; the bacterial contamination that affected the water of more than 30,000 New York City residents in July, 1993; and studies showing that chemicals such as chlorine, radon, and arsenic may cause cancer and birth defects.

Recently, a study, done by the University of Texas Medical School and released in the *New England Journal of Medicine,* revealed that cryptosporidium, the parasite, *". . . is common in water supplies, and can infect people at very low doses."* According to Dr. Herbert L. DuPont of St. Luke's Episcopal Hospital in Houston, *"Virtually anybody can be infected with this bug"* [emphasis added]. The disease can be dangerous, even fatal, to people with weakened immune systems. This "bug" is not killed by disinfectants and chlorination. In 1993, Oregon residents found their water riddled with asbestos; the EPA said that *30 million Americans* might be at risk from lead in their drinking water, and the National Resources Defense Council (NRDC) released a report claiming nearly *125 million Americans* should worry about the water they draw from their taps each day.

In a recent *USA Today* national survey, more than half the respondents said they were "very worried," and another one in four said they were "somewhat worried" about drinking water pollution.

In December, 1993, nearly one million people in the nation's capital and its suburbs were boiling tap water, clearing grocery shelves of bottled water, and keeping their mouths shut in the shower, following a federal warning that local drinking water may be contaminated. Officials announced the restriction out of concern over the possible presence at one of the reservoirs of a parasite that can cause intestinal illness. It was announced that the White House has its own filtration system and was not affected.

In October, 1994, a report released jointly by the Environmental Working Group (EWG), Physicians for Social Responsibility (PSR), and Citizen Action revealed, *"Over 14 million Americans* in the Chesapeake Bay region, the Midwest, and Louisiana face increased cancer risks from drinking water contaminated with widely used farming herbicides" [emphasis added]. The report states that water often is contaminated with two to four different herbicides at the same time. The cancer risks are 10 to 100 times higher than the federal benchmark, according to the report, especially in the Midwest. According to Richard Wiles, a vice president at EWG, "The drinking water in nearly every Midwestern city south of Chicago is contaminated with agricultural weed killers, and millions of Americans routinely drink water with unsafe levels of these herbicides." The EPA says the report should be viewed with concern but not alarm, but EPA Administrator Carol Browner admitted, "This study is another in a series of wake-up calls that tells us we can no longer take for granted that our drinking water is safe all the time."

The Environmental Protection Agency recently has estimated that about 19 million people across the United States are exposed to radon from drinking water at levels above its proposed maximum standard. Radon is a colorless, odorless, radioactive gas occurring naturally in the soil and ground water by decay of uranium and radium. When the water is used in a shower, a faucet, washing machine, or toilet, the radon becomes airborne, causing a health risk due to inhalation. *Radon is the second-leading cause of lung cancer in the U.S., only behind cigarette smoking.*

REGULATORY FAILURES

Another growing concern is that the regulatory bodies, whose responsibility it is to oversee water quality for consumers, *may be seriously deficient in their oversight responsibilities!*

The New York Times Magazine article referenced above also quoted a report by the General Accounting Office (GAO), Congress' investigative office, which says: "Small water system operators are inexperienced and under-trained, and more than 10 states actually exempt systems serving fewer than 500 people from operator certification requirements, *despite the fact that small systems account for 60% of the nation's water systems*" [emphasis added]. The GAO also criticizes many states for failing to conduct proper, timely water system surveys and inspections. A recent study by the National Resources Defense Council (NRDC) reveals, "Millions of Americans are exposed to health-threatening microorganisms and toxins because of *wide-spread and often undisclosed* contamination of drinking water" [emphasis added]. They point out that, ". . .despite massive numbers of violations of federal drinking water quality standards, water utilities face little threat of state or federal enforcement action."

Erik Olson, an NRDC attorney and author of the report, says, "Many utilities have capitalized on consumer faith and weak enforcement to let water quality slide."

The study revealed: more than *250,000 Safe Water Drinking*

Act violations between 1991 and 1992, affecting more than 120,000,000 people; nearly half of the U.S. community water systems violated SDWA standards, including more than 15,000 episodic or chronic violations of federal water quality standards affecting over 28,000,000 during the same period; non-community water systems, including hospitals, hotels, schools, and factories, were responsible for another 10,000 water quality violations, affecting 1,400,000 people; thousands of contamination incidents may be hidden from the public because of the 217,000 failures by water suppliers to comply with SDWA requirements to test water, report contamination events, comply with treatment techniques, and to notify the public of violations; *contamination problems are hidden from the public 63% of the time;* and even when violations are reported, enforcement action occurs in only slightly over 1% of the incidents.

The NRDC study also revealed that "...23 states inspect their water utilities less frequently now, than they were five years ago," and that "some consumers are drinking from systems that haven't been inspected in ten years."

If you think buying and drinking expensive bottled water provides the solution to this problem of contamination, this is not the case. The CBE Environmental Review refers to the bottled water industry as one "...*whose standards are no more stringent or no more rigorously enforced than those for tap water, and there is no assurance that bottled water is any more or less free from toxic chemical contamination*" [emphasis added].

Most bottlers are unable to provide a complete chemical analysis of finished water, and sanitary deficiencies are common in most all bottling facilities. *Warm temperatures speed up the growth of bacteria in bottled water sitting on the dealer's shelf. The longer it sits, the greater the risk!*

In a recent report issued by the U.S. Environmental Policy Institute, it was concluded, "In general, bottled water products are no safer or more healthful than most tap waters, and in fact, public water utilities are the source for over one-third of all bottled waters in the U.S." The report further disclosed that its product testing results show that bottled water "frequently" contains low levels of contaminants, such as heavy metals and solvents.

Based on the overwhelming body of scientific research avail-

able, it appears that the majority of water treatment plants are obsolete and incapable of solving the problems arising from dangerous chemicals, viruses, and metals now present in available source waters. If you drink the 6-8 glasses of water daily that your body needs, the evidence suggests you may be slowly poisoning your body and shortening your life. In addition, those responsible for protecting you apparently are fulfilling their responsibilities inadequately.

So, what is one to do?!?

HOME WATER TREATMENT THE ONLY SAFE SOLUTION

In recent years, millions around the world who share these concerns about the water crisis have sought to protect themselves and their families with home water treatment systems, as " . . . the only feasible way of ensuring that water is fit to drink." In the United States alone, *more than $1 Billion per year* is being spent for home drinking water treatment units and their replacement cartridges.

Bottled water still is used by 21% of households, *but nearly 30,000,000 Americans already have installed point-of-use (POU) or point-of-entry (POE) water treatment equipment.* Demand for bottled water has been flat for three years, and consumers are looking for a better, less expensive answer. These statistics recently were released as part of a 586-page report from Baytel Associates, a San Francisco-based market research and consulting firm specializing in water treatment markets.

Currently, about the same percentage of households use water treatment equipment that used garbage disposers or dishwashers in 1960. Between 1960 and 1980, one in three U.S. homes added a garbage disposer or a dishwasher. With the crisis in water, growth in water treatment systems can be expected to be much more dramatic.

A brief explanation of the two types of systems mentioned earlier is in order. A point-of-use (POU) filter is one that is attached directly to a faucet, most commonly at the kitchen and/or bathroom sink. It diverts the influent water into and through the unit which sits either on the counter (countertop) or under the sink (undercounter), and then routes the purified water to a faucet or spout for easy access.

The POU filter is suitable for filtering all the water you drink, cook with, mix flavored drinks with, or for making coffee, tea, juices, and washing fresh vegetables.

A point-of-entry unit is usually a "whole-house" system, placed near where the water enters the house or business, and provides treated water for the kitchen, the bathroom, the laundry, and anywhere else you use water within the structure.

When funds are limited, a point-of-use unit will solve perhaps the biggest immediate single problem, that of safe, clean water to drink and with which to cook. A modest additional investment into a quality shower filter designed specifically to remove the chlorine will solve the second biggest problem, that of showering and/or bathing in chlorine-treated or contaminated water.

The morning splash of a shower seems refreshing and invigorating, but if you're bathing in average American tap water, you're waking up to more exposure to water pollutants than you'll drink all day. According to the EPA, "THM's, formed when chlorine combines with the natural organic matter in the water, are present in virtually all chlorinated water supplies in the United States." Chloroform is the most common of the THM's and is known to cause liver and kidney damage and central nervous system depression, *and is a suspected human carcinogen*.

According to a study done by the Massachusetts Department of Environmental Quality Engineering, published in the May, 1984, issue of the *American Journal of Public Health,* " . . .20 to 46 percent of water pollutant exposure occurs through the skin in children and 50 to 70 percent occurs through the skin in adults. The actual amount varies dependent on the chemical and the concentration of the chemical in the water." A normal adult taking a 15-minute bath or shower each day would be exposed to up to *twice as much* of a volatile contaminant as from drinking two quarts of the same water! A child weighing 50 pounds would absorb *up to 10 times as much* contamination from swimming in a pool for an hour as from drinking a quart of the same water.

Researchers say that these figures are based on very conservative estimates, and they do not take into account a number of factors known to increase skin absorption, such as wetness of the skin, higher temperatures (such as found in a hot shower), breaks in the skin (abrasions, cuts, rashes, etc.), sunburn, and the use of soap. In addition, the data was based on experimental situations in which only the hand or thumb was immersed in the test solution.

The EPA study also discovered that THM's can escape from the water via mist and steam to become air pollution. They consistently found high levels of chloroform inside homes and concluded "the culprit was hot running shower water."

WHICH WATER PURIFIER IS BEST?

Choosing a home water purifying system can be confusing due to the several types and many brands offered. Each company claims theirs to be the best and parades the features and benefits of their units. We have been involved in the water purifier business since 1977 and have sold every type and many brands.

For many years, granular activated carbon (GAC) has been the most commonly used medium for home and industrial water filter applications, effectively removing chlorine, odors, bad taste, and color from tap water. Most water filter systems use GAC, even today. While GAC is an excellent means of organic pollutant removal, *it is unable to cope with bacteria problems.* In some instances, silver impregnation is utilized in an attempt to prevent the common problem of bacterial growth in the carbon filter, with questionable results. Granular carbon will remove chlorine, bad taste, odor, color, and organic compounds from water, but it is not effective against metals and other inorganic pollutants. Solid carbon block can remove some things that granular carbon can't. However, carbon technology, by itself, has become overwhelmed by the enormity of the contamination and pollution problems we face today.

Carbon remains an essential ingredient in water purification because of its unique pore structure and adsorptive quality. Because of the microscopic caverns throughout activated carbon, it is able to hold a great amount of contaminants. A small amount of activated carbon is equivalent to a large surface area. But to deal with today's level of contaminants, *carbon needs to be combined with other media.* For example, carbon combined with ceramic submicron filtration will accomplish much greater removal of contaminants than carbon alone, including bacteria, parasites, and the heavy metals. Many purists believe that distillation plus carbon, deionization plus carbon, or reverse osmosis plus carbon are the ultimate choices in purification.

Combining carbon with KDF (Kinetic Degradation Fluxion) represents *a major technological breakthrough in affordable water filtration systems,* and is perhaps the best industry news of this century. (More on KDF later.)

Distillation is the process of capturing recondensed steam from boiling the source water. It is essential to use carbon as a follow-up, especially with chlorinated water, because chlorine and some other chemicals in the water will be heated into gas and travel with the steam. The carbon will remove most of this chlorine and other volatile organics.

Deionization uses a resin to remove ionically-charged contaminants. It is also important to accompany the resin with carbon for the additional chemical removal that carbon provides.

Reverse Osmosis (RO) is a specialized type of screening of water contaminants. It utilizes a membrane of one or the other of two basic types: Cellulose Acetate (CA) or Thin Film Composite (TFC). *Osmosis* is a term you may remember from biology, referring to the passage of a substance through a membrane from a solution of greater concentration to one of lesser concentration. Reverse osmosis is forcing water under pressure through a membrane which excludes substances with a molecular structure larger than the pores of the membrane. A reverse osmosis unit operates from the source water pressure. A unique feature of reverse osmosis, compared with standard filtration methods, is that the molecules of water actually enter and become part of the membrane as they pass through. The membrane also allows oxygen through, as well as some other elements with a very small molecular size, including some colloidal minerals. The pores are small enough to screen out bacteria and even some viruses. Still, some small molecule contaminants can make it through, so a reverse osmosis unit always should include some type of carbon post-filter. Chlorine also can harm membranes. Chlorinated water requires a carbon pre-filter.

Both independent analyses and personal experience with the various methods of water purification lead us to the following conclusions:

The water resulting from distillation and deionization is so *devoid of mineral content* that it becomes aggressive in drawing up minerals. This can result in a significant mineral loss from the body, if not adequately compensated by adding supplementary minerals to the water or to the diet. Distilled water is also practically *devoid of free oxygen*, an important beneficial health factor.

Although reverse osmosis water actually has an increased oxygen concentration and contains small quantities of colloidal minerals, it also *is lacking in mineral value* and will draw minerals from the body. Furthermore, reverse osmosis units are *very susceptible to bacterial growth* in the system, especially when not in use. Bacteria can attack and ruin a membrane. A low bacterial count in the source water is important. Ideally, RO's work best when run constantly, which in most instances is neither practical nor economical.

There are those who would suggest that water is not a dependable source of all the minerals required for nutritional purposes, as the mineral content may vary from place to place, and even from the same source over time. This is true, however, many people get more mineral value from their drinking water than from their food intake today, because the agricultural soils are so overworked that they are seriously mineral deficient. Further, the body needs the colloidal minerals that are in the water to accomplish certain electrical transmissions throughout the system. *The net loss of minerals from the body due to consuming mineral-devalued water can have a significant long-term negative impact on health and longevity.*

For these reasons, *distillation, deionization, and reverse osmosis all have serious drawbacks.* More than this, distillation and reverse osmosis are both *inefficient* in their use of resources. Both waste a great deal of water in the process of their functioning. *Reverse osmosis wastes 4 to 6 gallons of water for every gallon of pure water produced.* This water flushes away the contaminants rejected by the membrane. Distillers not only waste water, but also require a great amount of electricity to operate. Deionizers, in addition, need to have their resin "recharged" frequently, a service for which there is a fee.

All three of these methods require frequent attention to maintenance. No purification method works well if not well maintained. This is most important, because if people do not keep up with replacement of exhausted pre-, primary- and post-filter RO membranes or deionizing resins, the water quality will be quite bad, often before it is recognized by the consumers. This is too often the case. Unfortunately, a proper schedule of replacement of water system parts is seldom followed.

A SIGNIFICANT BREAKTHROUGH

Recently (1987), an exciting new technological breakthrough for water filtration was discovered. Developed and designed by a leading American scientist, this new system, Kinetic Degradation Fluxion (KDF), has been awarded both U.S. and international patents.

KDF utilizes an all-natural process in which dissimilar metals are used to set up a kinetic charge that *kills* microorganisms and *alters or removes* many problem contaminants. It also *conditions* water with a "softening" effect, as it transforms the minerals into colloids, their most bioavailable and healthful state. KDF has been proven to be the *best way to remove major contaminants from our water, and shown to stay active longer than any other purification method.* In most cases, the result is better water than bottled water, at a fraction of the cost.

In August, 1992, KDF was awarded the U.S. EPA's approval as a "pesticidal device," which means it has the ability to kill algae, bacteria (including *Pseudomonas florescens, Ybrio cholera, Legionella pneumophilia,* and coliforms), fungus, mold, and many parasites and viruses found in drinking water supplies, through the natural process of *electrochemical oxidation/reduction.*

KDF also has been certified to kill a target bacteria within the "less than 1.0 minute contact time" required to be effective in point-of-use water filters. Thus it is "bacteriacidal," a much-preferred classification to that of "bacteriostatic," a term often used with silver impregnation which only slightly retards bacterial growth.

When this KDF technology is combined with high-quality coconut shell carbon, the result is truly revolutionary. The KDF protects the carbon from rapid exhaustion with chlorine by handling the chlorine first, thus allowing the carbon to have a much longer effective life. *KDF has TEN TIMES or more the life expectancy of activated carbon!* KDF and carbon, working together, have been proven effective against microorganisms, chlorine, heavy metals (aluminum, arsenic, cadmium, iron, lead, mercury, etc.), hydrogen sulfide, nitrates, odor, poor taste, THM's, PCB's, dioxin, and thousands of other organic chemicals and inorganic poisons...*at a cost of approximately one cent per gallon!*

WATER PROBLEMS AND TREATMENTS

This chart is compiled from information taken from various product brochures, technical books, information provided from the Water Quality Association and trade journal articles. Most information excludes percentages of contaminants removed and capacities of these systems to remove or reduce these contaminants. While much information we encounter represents different conclusions and opinions we felt these didn't reflect inaccuracies as much as they pointed out the complexities associated with treating water quality problems.

Problem	KDF & CARBON	DISTILLA-TION	Reverse Osmosis	Deionization	Ozone	UV	Cation Exchange	Anion Exchange	Chlorine	100% Carbon Filters	KDF/Carbon+Ceramic
Arsenic	■	■	■				■			□	■
Aluminum	■	■	■	■			■				■
Bacteria E. Coli-Pseudemonas	■	■	■		■	■			■		■
Barium	■	■	■	■			■				■
Cadmium	■	■	■	■			■				■
Chlorine	■									■	■
Chromium VI	■	■	■	■			■				■
Chromium III	■	■	■	■			■				■
Endrin	■		□							□	■
Fluoride	□	■	■								
Hydrogen Sulfide	■	■			■						■
Iron	■	■	■	■			■			□	■
Lead	■	■	■	■			■				■
Lindane	□		□							□	□
Mercury	■	■	■	■			■				■
Methoxychlor	■	■	□								
Nitrate (AS N)	□	■	■	■				■			■
Odor	■		□							■	■
Radon	■									■	■
Selenium	■	■	■					■			■
Silvex 2,3,5,-TP	■	■	□							□	■
Taste	■	■			□					■	■
Toxaphene	■	■	□							□	■
2, 4-D	■	■								□	■
THM's	■	■	■							■	■
TOTALS	25	20	20	9	4	1	9	2	1	12	25

Key ■ Effectively Removes   □ Significantly Reduces

CONCLUSION

While bottled water may be an improvement over chlorinated tap water, *any* on-site, well-maintained point-of-use or point-of-entry water purification system would be preferable to bottled water, which is considered by many to be unreliable.

With either POU or POE purification, you know what you are getting, and the cost per gallon is vastly lower than bottled water. This comparison should help clarify the relative merits and deficiencies of the various methods of water purification.

For the *health-conscious* individual who is also *cost-conscious* and prefers *long-term uninterrupted service,* the new **KDF/Carbon technology** offers the most attractive choice for *quality, value, and maintenance-free performance.* This would be true especially with modestly priced countertop and under-the-counter units.

For the ultimate in *affordable contaminant removal,* combining KDF with high-quality coconut shell granular activated carbon, plus ceramic technology, provides the best of all solutions...*all the quality water you want...when you want it...with an absolute minimum of service and maintenance.*

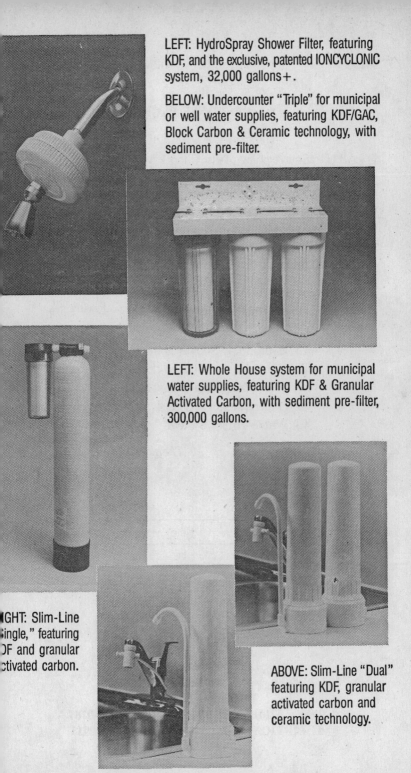

LEFT: HydroSpray Shower Filter, featuring KDF, and the exclusive, patented IONCYCLONIC system, 32,000 gallons+.

BELOW: Undercounter "Triple" for municipal or well water supplies, featuring KDF/GAC, Block Carbon & Ceramic technology, with sediment pre-filter.

LEFT: Whole House system for municipal water supplies, featuring KDF & Granular Activated Carbon, with sediment pre-filter, 300,000 gallons.

RIGHT: Slim-Line "Single," featuring KDF and granular activated carbon.

ABOVE: Slim-Line "Dual" featuring KDF, granular activated carbon and ceramic technology.

— RESPONSE PAGE —

All UltraSource point-of-use filters have replaceable cartridges and prices start at under $100.00. Prices for whole-house systems start at under $600.00. UltraSource honors VISA, MasterCard, and DISCOVER cards.

Dear Lyle and Jon,

I read about your water purification systems in Lindsey Williams' NEW book, *You Can LIVE!*

Please send me more information on the following:

        ☐ HydroSpray Shower Filter
        ☐ Slim-Line Countertop "Single"
        ☐ Slim-Line Countertop "Dual"
        ☐ UnderCounter "Triple"
        ☐ Whole-House System

Thank you!

PLEASE PRINT:

Name _____

Address _____

City/State/Zip _____

Telephone (_____) _____

Please make your selection(s) and send to:

UltraSource, Inc.
P. O. Box 237
Tallmadge, OH 44278
Phone: (216) 630-2700 • Fax: (216) 630-0787
TOLL-FREE Order Number 1-800-829-9913

Chapter 12

PHYTOPYC™
Nature's Warrior

By Anae Campbell
Sterling Health™ Marketing Group

A healthy body is the guest chamber of the soul; a sick one its prison.

The past 30 years have revealed not only an evolution in all standards of living, but an evolution in natural healing and alternative choices in the care of the human body. It appears the time is now to utilize the gifts of nature to their best effect. The greatest gifts are products untouched by man or technology.

Fall, 1995, witnesses the introduction by Sterling Health™ of a new product designed to awaken the immune system and integrate oxygen and nutrition to each cell. Unique to this formula is an ancient American Indian life-saving remedy for scurvy given to a group of French explorers in the 1500's, available now as PHYTOPYC™ (PHYTO—from plants; PYC— pycnogenols from grape seeds; nature's most powerful antiaging, antioxidants—50 times more powerful than Vitamin E and 18 times more effective than Vitamin C).

The ingredients of this supplement have been written on the walls of history. It contains the oldest healing known to man, that of essential oils. The essential oils are extracted carefully, keeping the high integrity of the total chemistry without bruising any molecule of the source. This gives exceptional healing to the human system by presenting each cell with the arterial life-force of the plant. Wholeness is made a reality and the body truly has an experience of its birthright, the celebration of living at the atomic level.

The mineral elements of this product are potassium, magnesium, and calcium. These are necessary builders of life and the systems they influence. Calcium and potassium in citrate form are more bioavailable than almost any other. Magnesium oxide is more water soluble than most other forms, meaning that the blood cell and nerve cell can utilize it faster and more efficiently.

In addition to the regulation of metabolism (described later in this chapter), calcium is vital in the formation of strong bones and teeth, important in the maintenance of regular heartbeat, the transmission of nerve impulses, muscle growth and contraction, and preventing muscle cramps. This important mineral is essential in blood clotting and helps prevent colon cancer. It may lower blood pressure and prevent bone loss. It participates in the use of protein digestion and assimilation, preventing the acids of poor assimilation from poisoning the system. The loss of calcium comes from eating too much sugar and by having too high a protein diet. Bed rest for long periods cause all the electrolytes to be flushed away. Standing weight is most important in the vitality of calcium to the bones. Calcium is involved in the activation of several enzymes, including lipase (digestion of fats).

Magnesium helps prevent depression, dizziness, muscle weakness, twitching, heart disease, and high blood pressure, and aids in maintaining the proper pH balance. A most important job of this electrolyte is its ability to enable utilization of calcium and potassium. Magnesium is responsible for reducing and dissolving calcium phosphate stones. It protects the arterial lining from stress and plays an important role in carbohydrate and mineral metabolism. Consumption of high amounts of alcohol and diuretics, diarrhea, and the imbalance of other minerals, such as zinc, can result in a deficiency of magnesium. Decrease in magnesium absorption may come from the consumption of large amounts of fats, high oxalic acid foods, such as almonds, chard, coca, spinach, and caffeine drinks.

It has been stated that more than 80% of Americans are

potassium-deficient. Potassium is needed for proper secretion of hormones. Hormonal deficiency is first a mineral deficiency. Due to the high stress of the American way of life, the hormone balance is disrupted, causing a decrease in the sodium-potassium ratio to the cell. This mineral helps prevent stroke, aids in muscle contraction, and works with sodium to control body-water balance. It is important for a healthy nervous system, a regular heartbeat, stable blood pressure, and the electrochemical impulses to transfer nutrients to the cells.

An important vitamin, heart-to-heart protector, is Vitamin E. It is an antioxidant which improves circulation, repairs tissue, and aids in the prevention of cancer and cardiovascular disease. Vitamin E also has been linked to lowering the risk of the most common of cataract formations. The nutrient may help by shielding the lens against oxidation damage, which may be caused by such factors as cigarette smoking.

A small pilot study suggests the nutrient may help the heart by slowing atherosclerosis. For 12 weeks, two groups of 12 normal men were given daily either 800 international units (I.U.) of Vitamin E or a placebo. In the men who received the Vitamin E, LDL cholesterol was 50% less likely to undergo oxidation. That is a process in which free-radical oxygen molecules cause the cholesterol particles to turn rancid. Researchers speculate that this, in turn, could lead to clogged arteries.

The body needs zinc to maintain the proper levels of Vitamin E in the blood.

The "antistress" vitamin, pantothenic acid, plays a role in the production of the adrenal hormones and formation of antibodies, aids in vitamin utilization, and helps to convert fats, carbohydrates, and proteins into energy. There are probably very few items in one's diet that do not contain this vitamin. It is required by all cells in the body and is concentrated in the organs. It is water- glycerin-, alcohol-, chloroform-, and ether-soluble, therefore, making it valuable in all chemical functions of the body. Pantothenic acid is needed for normal functions of the gastrointestinal tract and found to be extremely helpful in the prevention of depression and anxiety.

PHYTOPYC™ also contains two vital herbs which are helpful to the usage of all the accompanying ingredients. Butcher's Broom is good for all disorders of the vein and artery system, including hemorrhoids and varicose veins, plus obstruction of the urinary system. A mild laxative, not only for the bowel, but it also causes perspiration, assisting the elimination of toxins through the skin, the largest eliminative organ of the human body. It takes that tired heavy feeling out of the legs. The second vital herb contained in PHYTOPYC™ is yucca. Yucca was used first as a shampoo for the entire body by the Native Americans. It emulsifies toxic impurities, accelerates the breakdown of organic wastes, such as stored uric acid which creates sore joints and muscles with exercise and stress. It relieves the acuteness of arthritis, rheumatic, and gout pain because it contains a natural form of cortisone. Yucca strengthens the natural intestinal flora. The imbalance of friendly flora is the base symptom of much dis-ease in today's unhealthy world. There is much data to indicate the possibility that the overuse of antibiotics contributes heavily to this type of problem.

Before presenting the individual essential oils and their benefits to this new formulation, it is vital to stress the importance of replenishing the oxygen in the cells. Cell-anemia from insufficient oxygen is one of the basic underlying causes of poor health. The essential oils deliver oxygen to the cell in as efficient a manner as is available today.

The definition of oxygen, according to the *Webster's Dictionary* and *The Merck Index* is: a colorless, odorless, tasteless, natural gas; supports combustion. Is it not ironic how these major references (and five others on elemental nutrients and nutrition) do not mention oxygen as a life-sustaining substance? Even a kindergarten child knows the human, plant, animal, and mineral kingdom, water and the ocean world, the atmosphere—all forms of life cannot live without the presence of oxygen.

The lack of oxygen at cell level causes disease, thereby causing dysfunctional minds and bodies. The breath is directly responsible for the delivery of nourishment to the cell, giving energy and zest for living. Shallow, short breathing leads to body devitalization, chronic fatigue, low energy, and even mental depression. Apathy is the body's way of conserving energy when oxygen is not effectively present for the delivery of protein to the cell.

Oxygen is the most important element for assimilation of proteins. Protein malnutrition results in the disturbance of water balance (edema), reduced synthesis of key hormones (lower body temperature), lack of proteins to transport nutrients into and out of the circulatory system (anemia), lack of protein to carry oxygen to the cells (muscular weakness), or to carry out the carbon dioxide (sleeplessness), and lack of protein to build collagen for scar formation (poor healing of wounds), and for growth of bones and teeth (stunted growth).

A popular concern is a slim, trim body, free of lumpy cellulite bulges. Changing breathing habits to a full life-sustaining breath will oxidize the cellulite. Paying particular attention to breathing properly when at the beach is an advantage to the release of impurities because of the salty air.

The essential oils of fir, spruce, pine, oregano, and thyme are found in PHYTOPYC™. The pine family provides respiratory stimulants and expectorants. Expectorants encourage the loosing and subsequent expulsion of mucus from the system. The North American Indians used fir for medicinal and religious purposes. Pine will stimulate adrenocortical glands and is antiseptic to the liver and urinary system. Spruce oil is excellent for balancing the energy, and opening and elevating the mind and spirit. The pines are a decongestant to the lymphatic system. They are anti-infectious, antifungal, and antiseptic.

Pasteur believed that external agents such as microbes, spores, and viruses were the cause of disease. This became the basic assumption of official medicine. From there, much of medicine has been concerned with killing these causes. Little is known in the modern world of how to keep the body from hosting such problems. There are scientific studies, dated 1881, on different methods of measuring the antiseptic power—in direct contact or in the vaporized state— of oregano. The ancients often grouped different species under the name *oregano* and praised its benefit for respiratory diseases, ulcers, burns, and poor digestion. Oregano is anti-infectious, antimicrobial, antifungal, antivirus, antibacterial, and antiparasitical. Placed directly on warts and other herpes outbreaks, one can witness fast and powerful healing. Oregano has been found to be valuable for the nervous system, adrenal health, hypertension, and nervous exhaustion.

Another antimicrobial, antibacterial, fungicide, parasiticide, and vermifuge is thyme. Healing to the stomach, nervous system, respiratory, and colon, it helps relieve rheumatism, psoriasis, warts, and yeast and staph infections. Its vital energy holds a vast spectrum of curative power. Throughout history, thyme has been used widely for therapy for warming, stimulation, and cleansing properties, as well as aiding the healing of wounds, sore throats, rheumatism, arthritis, and gout. The expectorant action of thyme has been known to assist with pulmonary diseases, removing bronchitis, tuberculosis, and asthma.

Truly, this new product, PHYTOPYC™, offers rejuvenation, regeneration, and simply new life to the powerful vehicle called the human being.

Many trusted institutions are beginning to fail: educational systems, banking systems, and communication systems, among others. That failure leads to informational overload. War for breakfast, a murder trial for lunch, plane crashes, rape, and mayhem for dinner have become a steady diet.

Our great-grandparents did not experience these environmental overloads. Each overload creates a poison that is stressful to the human body. The foremost enemy of the human being is gravity. The second greatest enemy is stress. How can we "de-stress"? How can we "de-traumatize" our world without creating more trauma?

It is said if mankind experiences the same amount of stress in the next 10 years as in the past ten—just the same amount. . . not more. . .with no increase (even though humanity always does increase)—the human being will be extinct within 150 years. How do we say, "Whoa!"?

Minerals from the Great Salt Lake provide one remedy—a miracle, an experience of perfection, electricity, and vitality at the smallest molecular structure. The major salts of sea water, namely, sodium, potassium, calcium, and magnesium—combine with chloride, phosphate, and carbonate to provide the general matrix for cells. The enzymes and vitamins incorporate the trace elements into the cells. Ratio to ratio, mineral to mineral, sea water is the same as perfect blood plasma. Life in mammals begins by the fertilized egg floating in an amniotic solution identical to sea water.

The contamination and devitalization of food and water sources create a stress overload, preventing balance in the human system. Through this stress, the electromagnetic system has been altered to such an extent that many people are allergic to foods, distressed by refrigerator noise, electricity, and computer sounds, and experience environmental illness. Children are unable to concentrate and study because of poisonous odors in the walls and carpets. People in general are unable to digest and assimilate food. Unfortunately, the body will not produce the necessary enzymes for proper digestion, while simultaneously being assaulted by the constant negativity of the six o'clock news. We have stress upon stress.

Remove the water from the human body, reduce it to ash, and what remains consists of 12 basic elements and 72 minor elements. The 12 basic elements connect us on many levels of our being to the planet of our birth. The most concentrated mineral is sodium, the second is magnesium, the stress element necessary for the vibrancy of all tissue and particularly the electric brain. With magnesium, the brain is able to send messages through the nervous system to all parts of the body for rejuvenation, restoration, and general function. It is of utmost importance that we have sufficient magnesium. Magnesium stimulates magnetically the rhythm of our breathing and our heart. It is absolutely essential for the assimilation of calcium. I will resume the subject of magnesium shortly, after I interject some vital information on calcium.

Another type of stress to the body currently is being inflicted —not an emotional stress, but a physical stress. This has resulted from use of assorted minerals in an improper ratio, which creates an imbalance in the body. Of particular concern is the improper use of calcium; even when used as the only supplement an imbalance occurs. The proper ratio between one mineral and another is critical, i.e. magnesium to calcium, sodium to potassium, etc. These imbalances in the elemental kingdom allow disease. By using types of calcium that the body neither can assimilate nor utilize, calcium poisoning occurs. Poisoning of any kind induces trauma to the system.

Calcium, the most abundant mineral in the body, is one of the most misunderstood nutrients. Rather than experiencing a calcium deficiency, most individuals, in fact, already have excess calcium in their tissues which they are unable to utilize. Consuming unnecessary calcium accelerates the decline into slowed metabolism and old age. Contrary to popular advertising, the most important function of calcium is *not* the creation of bone tissue, it is the regulation of the metabolism.

Magnesium activates more enzymes in the body than any other mineral. It is intimately involved in the storage of sugar as glycogen in the liver and in its release into the blood for energy. The so-called balanced diet provides only about 25% of the amount required for good health. Magnesium is involved more in the energy-producing reactions of the body than perhaps any other mineral. It is the first nutrient to be lost during stress. Magnesium, along with calcium, is the shock absorber to the human system. It tends to make the personality more flexible. The personality shapes mineral patterns; the mineral patterns shape personality. Magnesium presents a strong relationship to the way the physical system uses calcium, potassium, and sodium. It is required for the body to manufacture protein, fat, and other essentials which make up cells and intercellular material.

The balance between sodium and potassium, and the exchange of them in every body cell, is of utmost importance to the state of our health and gives energy to our life. The sodium-potassium pump, present in every cell, regulates the control of blood pressure. Most Americans' diets are too high in the problem ingredient (sodium chloride) and too low in the good ingredients (potassium, calcium, and magnesium). A diet high in potassium is nature's way of controlling hypertension. However, a sufficient amount of sodium is vital to proper function of the adrenal glands. The adrenals—the fight or flight regulators—are used up daily through our stress.

Swelling (edema) in the body is *not* due merely to excess sodium, then remedied simply by removing salt from the diet. Deficiency of potassium causes the cell to swell, protecting itself from the sodium which has gone to its center.

A tense person uses up a large amount of their mineral supply, which leads to fatigue, further depleting the body. A tired person has to push harder, causing an even greater drain on valuable body resources. A fatigued brain charged with extra activity causes repetitious processing. This condition of low nerve-cell energy causes the billions of brain cells to grow weak due to demineralization. The human nervous-brain system can be compared with dams on a river. Small dams are erected all along the nervous system. One giant dam is found in the brain; this dam holds back and keeps in check the flow of nerve and thought impulses that, otherwise, would pour in upon the consciousness. The lower the smaller dams, the more water that rushes over.

Applied to the nerve cells, the lower the energy source, the greater the flood of impulses—desired or undesired—that gush over the brain. The less energy existing in the nerve cell, the more it becomes irritated. This leads to a fatigued brain and nervous system.

Phosphorus is just one of the previous minerals needed by the brain for its power and vigor. Others are iron, iodine, silicon, sulfur, magnesium, and manganese. All these work together in harmony with vitamins and amino acids to create a strong brain. Sea water contains these named minerals in perfect balance.

Minerals are the basis of vitality to essential organs in our physical systems. The blood and the bones both use calcium, regulated by the parathyroid. Many stresses cause imbalance of the proper relationship. Improper digestion often causes an acidic and inflamed stomach, stiffness, soreness, and tenderness of joints. Calcium assists the proper pH, neutralizing the over-acid condition and buffering the body's painful reaction. Recently, calcium, potassium, and magnesium citrates have been found to be more easily assimilated than any other food source.

All minerals work in harmony with other essential life-giving nutrients. A deficiency of one mineral may disrupt the entire chain of life, rendering other nutrients either useless or inefficient. The importance of the proper balance of minerals in the tissues and fluids of the body is very great. Any considerable departure from the norm is incompatible with life!

Dr. Carl Pfeiffer, author of *Mental and Elemental Nutrition,* reports in his book that in many cases of schizophrenia, there has proven to be a strong relationship of copper stability, Niacin, and Vitamin B6 to overall emotional health.

Another area of study shows the relationship of zinc to the immune system. Improper supplementation of zinc to the AIDS patient is detrimental and creates further poisoning. Zinc is important to the sense of smell, the sense of taste, and the repair of skin.

A highly questioned trace mineral supplemented medically for manic depression is lithium. Found in the balance of nature, it promotes a better attitude toward life. People in areas of America that are high in lithium are more relaxed and less aggressive. A study has been done that shows a correlation between a high crime rate and low lithium levels in the water.

Lithium's counterpart is rubidium. Rubidium is the Ponce de Leon fountain of youth element, inducing youthfulness, a pleasant attitude, and higher self-esteem, without aggression and anger. Vitality, energy, and enthusiasm can be experienced at the cellular level.

Ionic minerals from the Great Salt Lake offer the perfect health balance. Easily digested and assimilated to maintain a natural defense system, these trace minerals become beneficial in releasing many ailments. Many children who have been labeled "learning disabled" and "attention deficit" (ADD) are simply trace-mineral deficient.

The body-mind wants the body to be whole, well, and rejuvenated at all times. The intelligence says, "Heal thyself"— the ego says, "Survive." Science reveals that the cell can reproduce and repair itself in such a way that the human body could live 5,000 years.

Oriental medicine tells us that a toxic-free body is a disease-free body. A healthy body does not host parasites, viruses, bacteria, and toxins. To create healing, the body often will draw parasites and/or bacteria to digest the overloaded toxic condition.

Sterling Health/Marine Minerals is a pioneer company in developing and presenting supplements unique in their pristine pureness. They have developed several formulas based upon the principle of the natural minerals from the water of the Great Salt Lake. These formulations have been planned carefully and are designed using enzymes, vitamins, minerals, herbs, and essential oils—for maintaining a healthy, stable body.

Two particular formulas combined deactivate and unwind the stress of the day. Stress Free™ and Cell-lectric™ can address the brain stress of those professionals in high-pressure fields such as advertising, computers, systems designers, engineers, pilots, or any person having to use the electrical effect of their brain on a continual basis. It enables them to put the brain to bed and sleep restfully.

Not all aloe vera products are created equal. Sterling Health Aloe Maia™ is an authentic, organically grown, properly prepared aloe vera which has powerful healing properties. The whole leaf, cold-pressed product is superior to those containing only the gel because the outer leaf and rind are used, which contain more of the active therapeutic substances.

Increasing popularity in health and nutrition has brought awareness of the importance of antioxidants and the dangers of free radicals. Free radicals are atoms or groups of atoms that can cause damage to our cells, impairing our immune system and leading to infections and various degenerative diseases. Antioxidants, such as Vitamins A, C, and E, protect the body from free radical damage.

Pycnogenols (most potent from grape seeds) are 18 times more powerful than Vitamin C and 50 times more than Vitamin E. They are a special class of water-soluble bioflavonoids instantly bioavailable to man, and they are the strongest, most potent antioxidant, known in many parts of the world for their antiaging properties, systematically relieving stress, atherosclerosis, diabetic retinopathy, edema, inflammation, varicose veins, skin elasticity, and joint flexibility. Bioflavonoids are a group of low molecular weight plant substances with recognized antioxidant (free radical scavenging) properties with the ability to inhibit the activity of certain enzymes which cause inflammation in the body. The bioflavonoids that make up pcynogenols are special. They are called proanthocyanidins. Sterling Health pycnogenols contain only the original pharmaceutical grade standardized Oligomeric Proantho-Cyanidin (OPC) extract invented and patented by Professor Jacques Masquelier of Bardot, France.

Pycnogenols alone produce the following effects: strengthen collagen and vascular system; prevent vascular and cerebral accidents, cross blood brain barrier; repair inflamed tissue; improve circulation; relieve PMS; reduce edema; balance blood sugar; moisten skin; prevent fatigue; relieve hay fever, asthma liver disease, and kidney problems.

Health is a word taken from the Anglo-Saxon, *haelth,* meaning "whole," and health has been defined as the absence of disease or the freedom from pain. Many people are willing to accept such a limited and negative definition. They think they are healthy if they manage to stay out of hospitals and get along without the services of a doctor.

Such individuals do admit that now and then they may suffer from sinusitis, bursitis, neuritis, arthritis, indigestion, constipation, fluttering of the heart, high blood pressure, athlete's foot, fatigue, anemia, obesity, skin disorders, baldness, colds, decayed teeth, poor eyesight, assorted allergies, brittle fingernails, nervousness, and even occasional mental depression.

Many may not be really sick, but how many are really well, exuding well-being like an energetic child or puppy?

Most just accept these conditions as the inevitable signs of aging and take comfort in thinking that if things get too bad, a new miracle drug will take care of it. So they continue to overeat, oversmoke, overdrink, get too little rest and exercise, and ignore the future.

This is not a happy way to live. If one honestly can admit that they have even one of these ailments, then they must face the fact that they do not have complete mental and physical health.

Reference

Pfeiffer, C.C., *Mental and Elemental Nutrients*. Keats Publishing, Inc., Connecticut, 1975.

Anae Campbell

Anae Campbell has been studying, teaching, and counseling for 27 years in the fields of nutrition, herbology, iridology, natural healing, cranial sacral therapy, Amma Process, and other modalities. She is much in demand for private counseling and travels widely in the United States to present workshops. She has designed herbal/mineral formulas for the enhancement of general health and vitality. Her earlier years were focused on the successful therapy and healing in conjunction with her son, who suffered with cerebral palsy due to oxygen deprivation in post-natal care. This was her main motivation in becoming a full-time health practitioner.

— RESPONSE PAGE —

I read about your new supplement, PHYTOPYC™, in Lindsey Williams' new book, *You Can LIVE!* Please send me information on how to order PHYTOPYC™ and a catalog of your other supplements for good health.

Thank you!

PLEASE PRINT:

Name _____

Address _____

City/State/Zip _____

Telephone (_____) _____

For additional information, please contact the person who loaned you this book, or contact:

Sterling Health
2066 South 950 East
Provo, UT 84606
Phone: (801) 375-6590 • Fax: (801) 377-7999
TOLL-FREE Order Number 1-800-444-8077

Chapter 13

Family Preparedness, Health, and Survival Supplies

By Richard Mankamyer
The Survival Center™

The Survival Center™ is America's oldest continually operating family preparedness, health, and survival supply
company. We offer thousands of health and survival products
under one roof, more of them than almost anybody else—Food
(food supplies and equipment), heat, light, and power products
(alternative energy sources), health, security, and shelter items,
tools, books, videos, and much more, including two catalogs and
lots of valuable, necessary information.

With almost **25 years' experience,** The Survival Center™
offers a depth of knowledge and assistance not commonly found
elsewhere. We empower people to be able to care for themselves
and their families by successful preparation of the four basics
of survival: (1) food, (2) water, (3) medical, and (4) shelter.

We are highly dedicated and experienced people who practice
what we preach—*self-reliant living*—an idea that went out of
style in the past century. In recent years, self-reliant living once
again became fashionable. However, what used to be *trendy* is
now *necessary.*

We are located in the evergreen Pacific Northwest. We are as close as your front door and use UPS and other daily delivery services. Special reduced rates are available for heavier orders.

DID YOU KNOW?

1. "The No. 1 problem facing the world in the 1990's will be worldwide food shortages which will create a crisis of global proportions..." (1976 CIA Report).
2. Strange and unusual weather is being experienced all over the planet and storms are on the increase.
3. Earthquakes are more frequent and they are stronger.
4. Atmospheric CO_2 (carbon dioxide) is rising, threatening crop production and life on earth. From a low in the 1800's of 260 ppm to over 350 ppm in the 1990's, and rising.
5. Tornadoes increased in the USA some 350% between 1950-1986.
6. Plagues are showing up in many countries—some are airborne. Lack of proper food and nutrition contributes to the spread of disease.
7. World food consumption exceeded production in the late 1980's.
8. Each day, UNICEF estimates, 40,000 people starve to death, most of them children. $40,000 \times 365$ days a year $= 14,600,000$ die each year from the lack of food. This figure is rising.
9. When the climate changes and earth frequencies are altered, funguses, bacteria, viruses, and parasites mutate.
10. Food and water supplies could become contaminated by the various viruses.

WHY YOU SHOULD BE PREPARED!

Preparedness prevents panic. We help prepare people for emergencies and disasters. The more you are prepared, the less likely you will panic.

With many changes sweeping the land, life is becoming both challenging and, at times, precarious. Knowledge, protection of self and family, and health of the body are becoming more important than ever.

New diseases are rampant and the food supplies could become contaminated. Political intrigue increases. Land masses and weather patterns are shifting and changing erratically. All these factors intertwine to create an environment that potentially upsets the accepted balance of life as we live it.

So why should you be interested in us? *Experience!* More so than most anyone in this field. Our depth of knowledge and practical experience far exceeds any others we have encountered. We wrote the book on preparedness titled, *Basic Preparedness.* Second, *product variety.* Ours is the largest and oldest *continually operating* family preparedness, health, and survival supply center in the country. In addition to providing thousands of products for preparedness and survival, we also offer free food storage counseling and service that's quick, efficient, and friendly. We ship most items from our centrally located warehouses direct to all points in the continental United States, plus Alaska, Canada, and the rest of the free world.

You do have options. Whether you are a beginner or have some advanced experience at preparedness and survival, we can assist you in personalizing your needs, using our hands-on experience and expertise that spans almost 25 years.

Our prices are low because we buy in quantity, and we've been keeping them that way for a long time. We pass the savings on to you, our customers. The better prepared you are, the better off we all will be in an emergency.

In today's rapidly changing environment, emergency situations and disasters are making it necessary to have on hand a reserve supply of food, water, and daily essentials. It is necessary to prepare for situations where there will be loss of electricity, heat, and the ability to travel to the local store.

One of the *greatest problems* during natural disasters is the incredible *difficulty for emergency services to function as planned* and reach all the areas of emergency quickly and efficiently. Individuals and families often are left to fend for themselves, with no outside help except from their neighbors.

Indeed, we have a great deal to offer. Being interested in us is being interested in yourself and the quality of your life in days of change and challenge. We take a modern approach to pioneer attitudes of preparedness and self-sufficiency—which is one of the things that made this country strong. YOU NEED TO BE PREPARED NOW and *you need experts to help you.*

WE ARE THE EXPERTS

We have been in the business of preparedness and survival

supplies for almost **25 years**. We carry one of the greatest selections of preparedness supplies and books available anywhere. Over the years, people have searched high and low for basic information and help on how to prepare for emergenices and disasters. Our many years of practical hands-on experience, expertise, and knowledge have enabled us to put these basics into one powerful book that every family in America should have on their shelves, *Basic Preparedness*.

The Survival Center™ staff are considered experts on a wide variety of products and services. We consult with many governmental agencies in developing their preparedness programs. We assist businesses, families, and individuals in customizing preparedness and self-sufficiency according to personal needs and handle inquiries from all over the world.

We were one of the first, and are still one of the only ones to manufacture and sell an underground shelter.

We can help you with "what you always wanted to know about survival but were afraid to ask." If you don't know the first thing about survival and self-sufficiency, we want you to call us and get our catalog so you can see what *options* you have available. Let us help you get started today. We are the experts. *Consider us your personal preparedness consultants and call us today! Prepare because you care!*

OUR PHILOSOPHY

The Survival Center™ was founded in the early 70's by Richard Mankamyer. The original concept was to educate people to take responsibility for their life and become more self-sufficient, empowering them with the knowledge and resources to better care for themselves and their families. We began specializing in the areas of food storage, alternative energy, health, and the supplies and equipment to do so.

As the years have passed, The Survival Center™ has become the headquarters for an incredible range of options and information, an alternative outlet where one can buy the hard-to-find items needed to become self-sufficient and knowledgeable.

The primary aim was (and still is) to provide food storage—whole, unadulterated staple foods—and sell them at competitive prices.

The Survival Center™ currently stocks thousands of items

under the general heading of "Family Preparedness, Health, and Survival" and is constantly expanding supplies and resources. In addition to long-term storage foods (nitrogen packed, freeze dried, MRE's, and more), our items include health and nutritional supplements, books and video tapes, survival and defense supplies, alternative forms of energy, homesteading supplies, more books, emergency first aid and survival kits, and much more.

In addition to our basic Survival Center™ catalog ($2.00), we now offer a second catalog dealing with alternative energy, i.e. solar, wind, and hydroelectric power systems and its many applications, including back-up generators, batteries, etc. The Solar Electric catalog is $4.95. The book *Basic Preparedness* is $16.95. Available from: **The Survival Center™, P. O. Box 234, McKenna, WA 98558—Phone (360) 458-6778.**

The following pages list a sampling of the reference material, family preparedness supplies, and survival equipment available to assist you in becoming healthier, more prepared, and self-sufficient. You have options. Learn what they are and please. . . *Get Ready!*

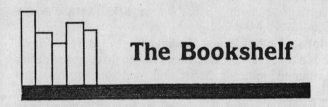

The Bookshelf

The following is a partial listing of some of the great books we stock at The Survival Center™. Empower yourself with the gift of knowledge. The more you know, the better you can make an intelligent decision. Build your library now. A more comprehensive list is in our catalog.

NOTE: Please add shipping and handling on all orders: Books— $2.50 for the first book; 95¢ for each additional book; Videos—$3.00 each.

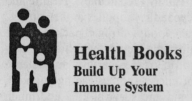

Health Books
Build Up Your
Immune System

A Holistic Protocol for the Immune System
The basic tenet of the holistic approach to medicine is that the body heals itself with some help. The author of this book feels, "Nature and the body have a wisdom that should be listened to; mankind should not immediately rush in with medical interference for every problem." If you are interested in a book that approaches AIDS, Candida, Hepatitis, and Chronic Fatigue Syndrome from a holistic viewpoint, this book is for you.   **BHF054 $15.95 + s&h**

The Handbook of Alternatives to Chemical Medicine
This book focuses on naturopathy through herbs, massage, nutrition, and other alternative methods. There are emergency procedures and approaches for whatever ails you, your pets, or your plants, from arthritis to worms. An excellent resource book.
                                        BHS012 $10.95 + s&h

Prescription for Nutritional Healing
This is a practical A-Z reference guide to drug-free remedies using vitamins, minerals, herbs, and food supplements. This book is in three parts. Part One explains the various nutrients and herbs available; Part Two describes common disorders from acne to cancer to yeast infection; and Part Three lists the traditional remedies and therapies most effective.
                                        BHF395 $16.95 + s&h

Healing with Whole Foods
Oriental traditions and modern nutrition. This book brings together authentic traditions of Oriental medicine with up-to-date research on healthy vegetarian diets, creating the ideal healing manual about food and its relationship to life.
                                        BHX046 $24.95 + s&h

Oxygen Healing Therapies

Scientists recognize that most disease states—including heart disease, cancer, immune disorders such as candida, and infection related to HIV—are caused by oxygen starvation at the cellular level. We receive most of our oxygen from the air around us, but breathing isn't always enough. Learn how to generate more oxygen in your body to achieve optimum health and longevity.

BHH609 $12.95 + s&h

Other outstanding books on the immune system.

Order No.	Title	Unit Price
BHH039	Alkalize or Die	$14.95
BHH106	Colon Health: The Key to Vibrant Life	5.95
BHH100	Echinacea: The Immune Herb	5.95
BHH026	Food: Your Miracle Medicine	13.00
BHG127	Healing Power of Herbs	12.95
BHH160	Immune Power Boosters	10.95
BHF103	Immune System, Your Magic Doctor	10.00
BHF452	Oxygen Therapies	12.00
BHX033	Parasites, an Epidemic in Disguise	7.95
BHH087	Strengthen Your Immune System	12.95
BHH066	The Anti-Oxidants	2.95
BHX107	Family Guide to Homeopathy	15.00

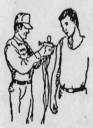

Immunization Awareness!

Immunization—The Reality Behind the Myth

The most up-to-date, completely and authoritatively documented, comprehensive critique of vaccines. From Pasteur's smallpox scam to vaccine-linked AIDS, this book is the state-of-the-art statement on vaccine damage. And its early chapters legitimately should terrify every parent whose child faces immunizations, as well as everyone who already has been so victimized.

BHF528 $12.95 + s&h

More important reading on immunizations.

Order No.	Title	Unit Price
BHS015	A Shot in the Dark	$10.95
BHX011	Immunization Decision—A Guide for Parents	8.95
BHH031	Vaccines: Are They Safe and Effective	7.95
BHH038	Vaccination and Immunization	13.95
BHH646	What Every Parent Should Know About Immunization	13.95

New Books and Videos

Order No.	Title	Unit Price
VIDCFC	VIDEO—The Cure for All Cancer	$19.95
BHH021	BOOK—The Cure for All Cancer	19.95
BHH178	BOOK—The Cure for HIV and AIDS	19.95
BHH609	BOOK—Oxygen Healing Therapies	12.95
BHH614	BOOK—The Un-Medical Miracle—Oxy	9.95
BUX040	BOOK—The Hot Zone (basis of movies like *Outbreak*)	6.99

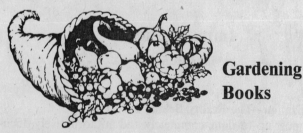

Gardening Books

Joy of Gardening

This book is the companion to the nationally acclaimed TV series featuring Dick Raymond. Full-color photos and illustrations and at-a-glance charts make Dick's proven methods

accessible to any gardener, beginner or seasoned expert.
                                        BGG017 $19.95 + s&h

The New Organic Growers' FOUR-SEASON HARVEST

The new organic growers' "*How To* harvest fresh, organic vegetables from your home garden all year long" book. Learn how to produce fresh, delicious, healthy food from your home garden year round. Be sure to get your copy of this invaluable resource.   **BGG025 $17.95 + s&h**

Perelandra Garden Workbook

"A complete guide to gardening with nature intelligences." This is a much-needed, hands-on manual for the gardener who wishes to work in conscious partnership with the overlighting nature intelligences. Truly a book for everyone seeking to connect into the larger picture of life.

                         Vol. I—BGX385 $19.95 + s&h
                         Vol. II—BGF115 $16.95 + s&h

The New Organic Grower

A master's manual of tools and techniques for the home and market gardener. "A welcome source of knowledge for anyone interested in small-scale, commercial farming and gardening without the use of harmful pesticides. Armed with cost-effective, environmentally sustainable production techniques presented in this important book, the grower can provide fresh produce we seek for our children and ourselves." **Meryl Streep** and **Wendy Gordon Rockefeller**, Co-Chairs, Mothers and Others for Pesticide Limits.   **BGG132 $19.95 + s&h**

The New Seed-Starters Handbook

For the most complete, up-to-date information on starting plants from seed, written by a gardener with 30 years' experience, this easy-to-use reference explains everything you need to know to start seeds and raise healthy seedlings successfully.
                                        BGG137 $15.95 + s&h

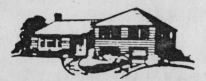 **Homesteading Books**

Finding and Buying Your Place in the Country

If you dream of "getting away from it all," make your dream come true—find your own place in the country! This "How To" book is a great resource. It walks the beginner through the process of buying rural land. It is well written, thorough, and up-to-date. Let this book help you make your dreams come true.

BDD015 $24.95 + s&h

Stocking Up, III Edition—The Classic Preserving Guide

This is one of our (The Survival Center's™) longest-running, most popular, "everyone should have it on their shelf" books we ever have sold. The most comprehensive, up-to-date guide to harvesting, storing, preparing, and preserving foods of all kinds. 627 pages full of helpful tips and stuff you need to know.

BDD091 $17.95 + s&h

The Encyclopedia of Country Living

No home is complete without this one-of-a-kind encyclopedia. For more than 20 years, people have relied on the hundreds of recipes, detailed instructions, and personal advice provided in this definitive classic. This book is about growing, processing, cooking, and preserving every kind of food—from the garden, the orchard, the field, or the barnyard. **BDX140 $24.95 + s&h**

Back to Basics—How to Learn and Enjoy Traditional American Skills

This book is a "classic" about the simple life. It is about old-fashioned ways of doing things and old-fashioned craftsmanship, food, and fun. It is about independence—the kind of down-home self-reliance that our grandparents and great-grandparents took for granted, but that we moderns often think has vanished forever. This is a "How To" book with hundreds of projects, step-by-step sequences, charts, tables, diagrams, and illustrations to help you and your family reestablish control over your day-to-day lives. **BDD020 $26.00 + s&h**

Other outstanding "How To" books on country living.

Order No.	Title	Unit Price
BBD465	Earthship Vol. 1—*How To* build your own house with old tires/cans, etc.	$24.95
BBD466	Earthship Vol. 2—More alternative *How To* ideas on building your own house	24.95
BBD467	Earthship Vol. 3—Latest research on alternatives to building your own house	24.95
BDD088	Root Cellaring—*How To* store your garden crops, etc. for the winter	12.95
BDD055	Foxfire Set, Vol. 1-9—Detailed *How To* information for home/farm	118.50
BBD014	Straw-Bale House—*How To* build your own house with bales of straw	30.00

 ## Alternative Energy Books

Living on 12 Volts with Ample Power

A must book for every user, builder, or technician of alternate energy systems. Learn how to store energy, how to produce energy, how to use energy, how to refrigerate. All design rules are explained with example so that you can buy or design your own Balanced Energy System.   **BED011 $25.00 + s&h**

The Independent Home

Living well with power from the sun, wind, and water. This "How To" book takes you inside the dwellings and lives of the renewable energy pioneers. According to the author, homeowners give up nothing, while they gain savings and independence. Hear it from the people who actually do it with alternative energy.
     BED010 $19.95 + s&h

Solar Electric Product & Planning Guide—132 pp.

This is not your ordinary catalog. We have included a great

deal of information, both on the products and how to use them.
The fast-find index gets you to your subject quickly and easily.
The planning guide starts from scratch, assuming that you know
nothing about solar power and electricity. From there, it advances
to explain the function of each component, and then how a
system is put together, giving examples of how others have done
so. Additional reference material also is available.

BED017 $4.95 + s&h

Other helpful books on Alternative Energy sources.

Order No.	Title	Unit Price
BED023	Wiring 12 Volts for Ample Power	$18.50
BED018	The Solar Electric House	21.95
BED022	Windpower for Home and Business	35.00
BED012	Living Without Electricity	5.95

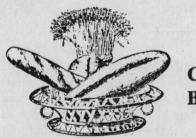

Cooking Books

The Bread Book—A Baker's Almanac
   This classic baking book has been a bestseller for over a decade
and a half. Learn *How To* make foolproof bread as a beginner,
time-saving tips for the busy baker, and many recipes for quick
breads, muffins, biscuits, and pancakes. Also includes a list of
bread-making supplies and equipment. **BCC011 $14.95 + s&h**

Sproutman's Kitchen Garden Cookbook
Sprout breads, cookies, soups, salads, and 250 other low-fat,
dairy-free, vegetarian recipes. 320 pages of exciting and different
ways of eating.   **BCC053 $14.95 + s&h**

Cooking with Home Storage

A delightful and informative cookbook written for those people who are looking for help in using their food storage. A collection of over 700 food-storage recipes, including many authentic pioneer recipes. Learn *How To* use dehydrated foods and make home remedies like Grandma used.

BCC212 $14.95 + s&h

New Laurel's Kitchen

A handbook for vegetarian cookery and nutrition. This book has been around almost as long as The Survival Center™. We have been selling this book ever since it was first printed back in the '70's. It includes over 500 recipes, ideas, menus, and suggestions, each tested and perfected for satisfying, wholesome home cooking. Highly recommended.   BCC045 $24.95 + s&h

Other wonderful cookbooks.

Order No.	Title	Unit Price
BCC037	Laurel's Kitchen Bread Book	$19.95
BDD075	New Concepts in Dry Food Cookery	12.95
BCC039	Moosewood Cookbook	11.95
BHC601	Recipes for a Small Planet	5.95
BHC015	Book of Whole Grains	4.95
BCC006	Back to Eden Cookbook	4.50

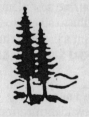

Survival Books

Where There Is No Doctor

A village health care handbook. Written for the Peace Corps and other places where medical facilities are not available. It explains in simple words and drawings what the average person can do to prevent, recognize, and treat many common sicknesses,

plus a lot more. This is one we all need to have on our shelf.
BHS235 $13.00 + s&h

Where There Is No Dentist
This is a companion to the village health care book, *Where There Is No Doctor.* Learn *How To* diagnose and treat dental problems, as well as help people care for their teeth and gums. Treatment and prevention is the main theme of this book.
BHS122 $6.50 + s&h

Basic Preparedness
This is an emergency preparedness manual that teaches you *How To* prepare for most anything that threatens your survival. The first four chapters cover the Four Basics of Survival (food, water, medical, shelter), and then expands into chapters covering grain usage and storage, food processing, homesteading, alternative energy, self-defense, and sovereignty. Also learn *How To* prepare and preserve food. Learn *How Much* food to store and *How To* create the most basic household products naturally.
BSS001 $16.95 + s&h

The Complete Wilderness Training Book
Field skills for adventures in the outdoors. Hundreds of useful skills for living off the land and surviving in the wild—even in the most adverse conditions. Learn *How To* build a lean-to-shelter, foliage bed, choose a campsite, dig a latrine, test plants for poison, gut a fish, make a compass, predict the weather, cross a fast river, signal for help, build a fire, and splint a broken arm. Includes many color photos and drawings. **BSS343 $29.95 + s&h**

How to Disappear Completely and Never Be Found
Planning a disappearance, arranging for new identification, finding work, and more. This book is for everyone with a need to not only disappear from their former life, but to start a new one. It tells *How To* plan a disappearance, document a new identity, find a job, and establish credit, plus coping with the crucial first few days, and more.   **BSS134 $6.95 + s&h**

Other vital books to help you survive a wilderness experience.

Order No.	Title	Unit Price
BSS523	Instant Guide to Edible Plants	$ 4.99
BS1009	Instant Guide to Medical Plants	4.99
BSS117	SAS Survival Manual	26.95
BSX044	Beginners Guide to Family Preparedness	10.95
BSZ021	How To Survive Without a Salary	12.95

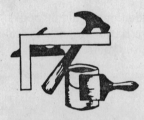

Building Books

The $50 & Up Underground House Book

This is a *How To* design and build underground book. Learn *How To* design an underground home. Get light, air, and views. Cut material cost up to 90%. Build greenhouses into the home. Build-in root cellars, fallout shelters. Use solar energy. Use hillsides. Solve drainage problems and deal with the building codes. Build a home from $50 to $15,000. **BBS127 $13.95 + s&h**

Building Small Barns, Sheds & Shelters

Extend your working, living, and storage areas with low-cost barns, sheds, and animal shelters. This book provides basic, easy-to-follow construction methods for attractive outbuildings. Here's complete information on tools and materials; foundations and floors; framing, sheathing, and roofing, plus windows and doors, wiring, and plumbing details. Specific plans and how-to-build instructions included.   **BBS905 $12.95 + s&h**

Shelters, Shacks, and Shanties

One of the great classics of outdoor lore. It is a complete guide to building all kinds of simple shelters, from the primitive Indian lean-to to the American log cabin. 300+ illustrations and step-by-step instructions for dozens of projects. **BBS097 $8.95 + s&h**

Other assorted building project books.

Order No.	Title	Unit Price
BBD458	Building a Solar-Heated Pit Greenhouse	$ 2.95
BBS112	Build Your Own Underground Root Cellar/Storm Shelter	2.95
BBS125	Building with Junk	19.95
BBS708	Build Your Own Low-Cost Log Home	12.95

See "Homesteading" section for additional building books. The Survival Center™ catalog lists over 1,000 titles of hard-to-find books. Be sure to get a catalog for yourself.

BASIC PREPAREDNESS
A Guide to Preparedness and
Self-Reliant Living

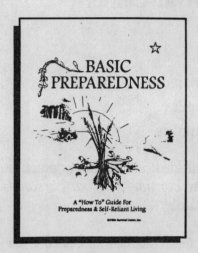

This is an *Emergency Preparedness Manual* that teaches the reader **How To** prepare for anything that threatens their survival. The idea of preparedness is spreading rapidly among those *waking up* to the reality of today's chaotic economic, geologic, and political climate. There are many reference books available that deal with specific areas of preparedness for an uncertain future. That's the problem. There are too many books. Most of us are busy and our reading time is precious. The *Four Basics* for successful survival are **food, water, medical, and shelter. This** *How To* book addresses all of these needs in the first four chapters, with easy-to-understand, simple instructions. Then the following chapters cover the basics of shelter, grain usage and storage, food processing, homesteading, alternative energy, self-defense, and sovereignty, plus an index and glossary. *Learn how to prepare for anything that could threaten the survival of you and your family.* Learn how to maintain a comfortable survival, regardless of the future situation. Learn how to prepare and preserve food. Learn *how much* food to store and how long it will keep. Learn how to create the most basic household products naturally. Learn how to set up your homestead to *run without power and still be comfortable.* Learn how to secure a piece of property that will shelter and feed your family, plus many more basic preparedness tips.

BSS001 $16.95 + s&h

— RESPONSE PAGE —

The Survival Center™

Your specialists in...

- Family Preparedness Supplies
- Health Supplies
- Survival Supplies

Our staff is knowledgeable, dedicated, and we "practice what we preach." *Please consider us your personal "Preparedness Consultants."*

If you would like to order from The Survival Center™, you may use your VISA or MasterCard and call us **Toll Free at 1-800-321-2900**, or Fax us at (360) 458-6868. For inquiries or general information, call us at (360) 458-6778 or write to:

The Survival Center™
P. O. Box 234 • McKenna, WA 98558

Be sure to mention that you read about us in Lindsey Williams' new book, *You Can LIVE!*

Thank you!

PLEASE PRINT:

Name _____

Address _____

City/State/Zip _____

Telephone (_____) _____

Chapter 14

Eating Out of Heaven's Garden

By Teri Williams, Joy of Living Health Seminars

Are you a person who really doesn't like to cook, or perhaps never really learned how to cook—but suddenly feels a need to eat better for the sake of your health? If you feel you are too old to learn or it is hopeless...*do not despair!*

I am probably the only daughter of a French chef who did not learn to cook until I was 35. If there is hope for me, there is hope for anyone. It's true! My dear mother, founder of *La Petite Ecole* French Cooking School tried everything possible to get me into the kitchen when I was young. However, I was such a tomboy that she could not keep me inside long enough to learn anything about cooking—except how to be a great "eater."

It was the day our first child was born when it hit me like the proverbial "ton of bricks"...I am responsible not only to feed this child, but to nourish her to health and maturity, and to do it according to the ways of our Heavenly Father. With the conviction brought about by this helpless baby in my arms, I began that very day to read every health food book I could find. I went to cooking classes, learning from everybody I knew who was committed to health—especially my husband Lindsey, who was patient and encouraging to me, as he had been eating healthy, whole foods for over 20 years. Finally, I went to the greatest source book ever written on this (or any other) subject, God's own Word.

So, these recipes are dedicated to all of you to whom cooking and eating whole foods is foreign or challenging. May you be encouraged and blessed for your efforts and desire to begin eating out of "Heaven's Garden" and giving the very best to your families.

We all know many reasons *why* we should eat healthy, but many of you may be wondering *how* to eat healthy. The most frequently-asked questions in my Joy of Living Health Seminars are: "Where do I start?" "How do I change life-long eating habits?" and "How do I even know what to buy at a Natural Foods Store?"

Our bodies became out of balance one step at a time, so let's put them back one step at a time. Once you know deep in your heart that God's plan for you and your family is to enjoy long years and good health, you already have crossed the biggest hurdle. Next, you just need to train your body to do what your mind and heart know is right. That's a bit tricky because you can expect your taste buds to make a giant protest! They have been feasting on sugar, salt, chemicals, caffeine, and fat for years—and loving every minute of it—as each of these items is very addictive. On the other hand, as we suffer more aches and pains, our bodies are begging for relief and help!

Well, let's start by taking away those tantalizing temptations. It's time to say a last "Good-bye" to all the foods in your pantry which are harmful, then replace them with foods which will nourish, sustain, and "love" you and your family.

It's as easy as one, two, three. First, *become an expert label reader.* Go through your pantry and begin reading the labels of everything you have. As you discover what is in most packaged foods (mostly words you cannot pronounce), you probably will do what I did...scream! Please, please—eliminate these from your shelves. You and your family deserve better. By eliminating the dead and harmful foods from your home, you make space for the life-giving foods your bodies need. Also, much of the "cravings" you experience is merely your body trying to tell you that it is not receiving some type of nourishment it requires. As you begin restoring it with *live* foods, gradually many of those cravings will leave you quite naturally.

Now that you have cleaned out your cupboards, you are ready

for the fun part—*stocking your kitchen naturally.* Going to a health food store for the first time may be a little intimidating because for years society has told us that junk foods are normal, and that natural foods are *strange.* All we have to do is look at the overall state of health of our national population and it is evident that the advertising is false. Please do not feel badly if anyone makes fun of you for eating healthy. Unfortunately, they are the losers. As is always the case, God gives us the final word of authority on the subject: "My people are destroyed for lack of knowledge. . . " (Hosea 4:6).

Today the choice of products available in health food stores is enormous, so your first trip can be overwhelming. Below is what I call the "Basic Starter Kit" for those who want to begin stocking your kitchen with healthy, natural commodities. It does require a small initial financial investment, but you will be able to prepare many of the recipes that follow with just these ingredients, and you can increase the variety of your "stock" as you go along. I also have included a list of brand names that I highly recommend. Our family has used their products over the years and found them to be good quality, pure and consistent. There are many other good brands available, as well, however these are the ones we personally use on a daily basis. I hope this list is helpful as you put together your Starter Kit.

BASIC STARTER KIT

Lots of organically-grown fruits and vegetables in season
Locally-raised organic eggs
1 bottle cold-pressed sesame or safflower oil
1 bottle extra virgin olive oil
1 pkg. 10-grain pancake mix, for rushed days (Bob's Red Mill is excellent)
1 or more boxes unsweetened breakfast cereals for children on rushed days
1 jar pure unsweetened jam or jelly
1 lb. freshly-made nut butter (peanut, almond, cashew, etc.), with no sugar
1 bag whole wheat flour
1 bag whole wheat pastry flour
1 bag organic unbleached flour
1 bag brown rice

1 bag whole oats
1 bag dried beans of your choice
1 qt. raw milk, or pasteurized only milk (no homogenized), or soy, rice, or almond milk
1 lb. raw unsalted nuts of your choice (roasting them at home is healthier)
1 lb. raw unprocessed honey grown in your region
1 of the following natural sweeteners: FruitSource®, Sucanat®, corn and barley malt, or stevia (stevia is especially good for anyone who is diabetic)
1 shaker of "real salt" or sea salt
1 pt. raw apple cider vinegar
1 qt. carob soy milk for children, instead of chocolate milk
1 or more (lead-free) cans of Sheldon's all-natural chicken broth
1 or more (lead-free) cans of Muir Glen organic crushed tomatoes
1 or more qts. unsweetened juices of your choice
1 or more lbs. Coleman's organic meat products, if you eat meat
1 or more lbs. Sheldon's poultry products, if you eat meat
1 or more lbs. raw milk cheeses, if you eat dairy
Panda brand all-natural licorice for children
1 small container non-aluminum baking powder
1 container Eden's brand Sesame Shake for seasoning rice, vegetables, and more
1 Bioforce brand "Herbamare" (season everything with it, including salad dressings)
1 Bragg's brand Aminos (flavor like soy sauce or tamari sauce, without fermentation)
1 Meyenberg brand goat's milk for children allergic to cow's milk

Several months later, try some variety—for example. . .other grains, such as millet, quinoa, amaranth, barley, and teff; other seeds, such as sesame, sunflower, pumpkin, and even sprouting seeds, such as alfalfa; other flours, such as barley, millet, soy, rye, and quinoa.

FAVORITE BRAND NAMES

Arrowhead Mills: organic grains, beans, cereals, and much more
AltaDena: dairy products, raw cheeses, cream cheese, honey ice cream, etc.

Barbara's: naturally-sweetened breakfast cereals, healthy snacks, cookies, etc.

Bioforce: Swiss seasonings; Herbamare

Brown Cow: pure yogurts

Cascadian Farms: pure, unsweetened jams, jellies, nut butters, organic frozen vegetables

Coleman's: clean meats

Earth's Best: organic baby foods and baby cereal

Eden: soy milk products

Fearn's: all-natural cake mixes

Frontier: dry herbs, vanilla without alcohol which has a superior flavor

FruitSource® : natural sweetener made from grape juice and whole rice syrup

Hain's: cold-pressed oils, healthy mayonnaise, etc.

Jensen's: broth seasonings, sweet whey powder, and much more

Knudsens: unsweetened juices

Meyenberg: goat's milk, for children who cannot drink cow's milk

Muir Glen: organic tomato products in lead-free cans

Panda: all-natural licorice

Santa Barbara: olives produced without chemicals

Santa Cruz: organic apple sauce

Sheldon's: clean meats

Spectrum: pure, cold-pressed vegetable oils and more

Sucanat® : natural sweetener from raw sugar cane

Since we all seem to have been born with a "sweet tooth," it is especially important to familiarize you with two of the most recent sources of sweeteners that are totally natural, healthy, and safe to feed to your family (in moderation, of course—obviously, too many sweets are not good for us). I have located two extremely reliable sources, and I wish space allowed me to duplicate all their wonderful material in this book; unfortunately, that is not the case, so I have paraphrased much of it below and sincerely suggest that you write the addresses I have furnished to request information about their products. They will happily furnish you with literature on research, statistics, nutritional content, and even some great recipes on how to use their products in some wonderful desserts.

Here is some of what FruitSource® has to say about its
product. "**Nature's Answer to Sugar:** FruitSource® Brand
Sweetener is pleasant-tasting, 100% natural and sugar-free;
newly-patented, made from grape juice and complex carbohydrates (whole rice), ideal alternative to refined sugar, artificial
sweeteners, and sugar substitutes. **Sweet Taste:** tastes like sugar;
none of the unpleasant aftertaste found in substitutes and
artificial sweeteners; no artificial flavors or colors; no preservatives; no refined sugar. **Lower Fat/Fresher Taste:** superior
moisture-retaining properties, which means up to 50% less salt
and fats and oils needed in baking; baked goods stay moist and
fresh-tasting longer. **All Purpose:** ideal for cooking, baking, and
everyday use; available in granular and liquid forms."

Of course, they guarantee your satisfaction and have a whole
array of helpful hints for using their product in your favorite
recipes, as well as tips on low-cholesterol cooking, and they invite
you to share with them some of your recipes using their product.
Address your inquiries to: FruitSource® Associates, 1803 Mission
St., Ste. 404, Santa Cruz, CA 95060.

The other sweetener I recommend is called Sucanat® . They
have produced an excellent article on sweeteners in general,
including the history of sugar as we know it today and why it
is harmful to our bodies. Titled "SUCANAT,® Nature's Original Sweetener: The End of the Sugar Blues," it is extremely
informative, and I suggest you write for a copy and study it
thoroughly: Pronatec International, Inc., P. O. Box 193, Peter-
borough, NH 03458, Phone (603) 924-9452.

Dr. Max-Henri Beguin, a Swiss pediatrician, became concerned about the effects of sugar on the health of his young
patients, not the least of which was tooth decay. In his research
he discovered that the problem was not with sugar, but rather
with *refined* sugar. "Complete" sugar, with all the nutrients still
in it, seemed to aid health and inhibit tooth decay. I have taken
the space below to reprint their chart, "Comparison of Nutrients
in Sweeteners," as I find the results astounding.

Sucanat® was fifteen years in the making. I quote a portion
from the article: "From the beginning, Dr. Beguin knew exactly
what he wanted. What was most elusive was the precise variety
of cane that would yield the most nutrient-rich, flavorful sugar;
a cane that was grown without chemical fertilizers or pesticides;

COMPARISON OF NUTRIENTS IN SWEETENERS
(All measurements one cup volume)*

	Sucanat 150g	Brown Sugar 150g	White Sugar 150g	Maple dried 150g	Honey liquid 339g	Malt dried 150g
Water	2.7g	2.1	0.4	2	17.2	28
Calories	570g	557	578	530	1031	557
Protein	1.05g	0	0	0	1.0	2.0
Carbohydrate	141g	144	140	137	279	117
Fat	0g	0	0	0	0	2.7
Sodium	0.5mg	45	1.5	21.4	17.0	23
Potassium	1125mg	514	4.5	370	173	348
Vitamin A	1600IU	0	0	—	0	—
Vitamin C	49.5mg	0	0	—	3.0	0
Thiamin (B1)	0.21mg	01	0	—	.02	.75
Riboflavin (B2)	21mg	04	0	—	.14	.48
Niacin	.20mg	0.3	0	—	1.0	13.9
Calcium	165mg	127	0	220	17	75
Iron	6.5mg	5.0	2	2.1	1.7	5.9
Vitamin B6	60mg	-	—	—	.07	—
Phosphorus	48mg	29	0	16	20	445
Magnesium	127mg	--	--	--	—	—
Zinc	2.3mg	—	1	—	—	—
Copper	0.3mg	—	—	—	—	—
Pantothenic Acid	1.8mg	--	—	—	—	—
Chromium	40mcg	--	--	—	—	—

Sources
USDA Handbook of Nutrient Content of Foods
Cantonal Laboratories of Zurich, Neuchatel, Valais and Basel, Switzerland
SpectroChem Laboratories, Franklin Lakes, N.J., U.S.A.

All values are averaged
* Please note: This is not a serving size, but a standard unit of measurement for comparing foods
- No data available

and a process that would retain all the vitamins and minerals that truly distinguish complete sugar from refined white sugar. The reason that organically-grown cane was of such fundamental importance was that with the minimal processing Dr. Beguin had conceived for his sugar, the final product would be highly concentrated. And a concentration of harmful chemical residues was absolutely out of the question. . . . Dr. Beguin searched the world over for years, pursuing one promising lead after another, until he found what he required. His perseverance finally was rewarded. Only developing a new and unique process for making complete sugar remained. The delicate balance of combining an advanced yet appropriate technology was the task of Pronatec (for Pro Natural Technologies)."

"Complete" sugar seems to be the answer, and the chart above certainly details why.

NOW, LET'S GET COOKING!

If you are not inclined to enjoy cooking, you may be thinking, "Spare me—I'll do it for my health, but I won't enjoy it!" Exactly what I thought! However, to my utter amazement, once I started "nourishing" my family, instead of just "feeding" them, a whole new feeling of gratitude and satisfaction slowly emerged in my heart. Suddenly, I had a greater appreciation for each of the foods that our Heavenly Father has created for us. As we began eating foods in their most natural state possible—the way they come right off the tree and right out of the garden, in season— everything began to have more flavor. We also increased the amount of raw foods we were eating, which immediately gave us all an increase in energy.

But the biggest reward of all has been our healthy children. I say this with all humility because Yaweh gets all the credit for helping us, although, I'm sure that *eating* healthy has played a major part in keeping them healthy. I can't remember the last time they had to see a doctor. With so much sickness all around us, we are thankful that the children have been spared much of it. Their healthful diets help them to have the stamina to resist much of the illness that is going around.

In today's kitchen, most of us have more gadgets than we can count. Before proceeding with the recipes, as a chef's daughter, I would like to share what I consider to be the only four items that one *really* needs to be a good chef. And if the term "chef" is somewhat intimidating to you, just call yourself a "loving cook." The first is a good paring knife, then a "French Chef" knife for cutting vegetables. The knives must be of utmost quality and kept very sharp. A sharp knife is much safer than a dull knife. (Saladmaster makes one of the best knives on the market, and they are lifetime guaranteed.) Next is a good, high-powered blender (we use a Vita Mix). Finally, you will want a good quality mixer for cookies, cakes, and bread making. The rest of the kitchen gadgets are optional, but really not necessary.

I believe one of the reasons that Americans eat far too few vegetables is because they never have been taught how to chop them quickly and efficiently. If you will take the time to learn to cut vegetables very fast and safely with your French Chef knife, I think you will be amazed at how much fun it is to prepare fresh vegetables, instead of frozen or canned ones. If necessary, invest in a cooking class just to learn the technique. It is worth gold to learn the art of cutting and preparing fresh vegetables. Our daughter, Elizabeth, has been chopping vegetables with a full-size French Chef knife since she was four years old! If she can do it, you and your children can, as well.

The following recipes are some of our family favorites. Many of them are very quick to prepare, which is a matter of concern for working mothers. The vegetable and meat pies take longer to prepare, but children and company just love them. Once you get the knack of doing a pie crust, you will love the results.

Happy Cooking...and most of all *very happy and healthy eating to you!*

Teri Williams

Teri Williams is the wife of author Lindsey Williams. She is the president of Joy of Living Health Seminars, coauthor of *Where's the Food?*, international lecturer on natural health, and "most important of all," according to Teri, the mother of two young children.

BREAKFAST IDEAS

1, 2, 3, 4, 5 Smoothie!

1 lg. banana	4 Tbsp. unsweetened plain yogurt
2 c. unsweetened apple juice	5 or more ice cubes to taste
3 sm. peaches	

Blend all ingredients in your blender on high speed. Scrumptious! Serves two or three.

Breakfast Energy Shake

2 c. unsweetened apple juice	1 handful raw unsalted almonds
½ c. frozen blueberries	1 handful raw unsalted sunflower seeds
½ c. frozen strawberries	
2 frozen bananas (remove peel, cut into pieces, and freeze in a zip lock bag)	4 heaping Tbsp. plain, unsweetened yogurt

Combine ingredients in a high-powered blender on high speed
for five minutes. Makes a rich, irresistible creamy shake. Serves 4.
(The reason for using frozen fruits is to get a nice cold shake.
If you use fresh fruits, add lots of ice.)

Summertime Fruit Plate with Yogurt and Nuts

At first glance, this may not sound too exciting. But when
arranged beautifully on a plate using fresh, ripe, organic fruits,
the flavor is outstanding!

1 apple	1 handful dried fruit, such as
1 peach	apricots or pears
1 pt. organic berries	1 handful chopped raw nuts of
1 banana	your choice
1 ripe avocado	1 c. plain unsweetened yogurt

Serves two. Use two large plates and two small bowls. Place one
bowl in the middle of each plate. Put yogurt in the bowls and
top with the fresh berries. Cut and arrange the fruit in a colorful
manner all around the plate. Sprinkle the nuts on top. Then serve
with a slice of whole grain bread and a nut butter of your choice.
Surprisingly elegant and delicious!

Potato Pancakes with Apple Sauce

3 potatoes, left over from last	¼ to ½ c. whole wheat flour to
night's dinner	make consistency of pancake
2 eggs	batter
1 tsp. baking powder	dash of garlic powder
	¼ tsp. Herbamare seasoning

Grate potatoes. Mix all ingredients; oil or butter your griddle.
Cook pancakes a little longer than regular pancakes, as they are
thicker and you want the egg to cook thoroughly. Garnish with
homemade apple sauce or Santa Cruz organic apple sauce and
a little pure maple syrup. This is a breakfast favorite in Germany.

Simple Vegetable Omelet

4 organic eggs	2 Tbsp. unsweetened plain
1 green zucchini	yogurt (optional)
¼ red pepper	1 Tbsp. fresh parsley
1 green onion	¼ c. grated raw cheddar cheese

Put small amount of butter or olive oil in your frying pan and heat up. Chop green onion and saute with sliced zucchini and small sliced red peppers until tender. In a separate bowl stir your eggs, using a wire wisk, then add the yogurt and other vegetables. Coat the bottom of your frying pan with a liquid lecithin and oil mixture (see recipe below) and heat. Pour in your egg/vegetable mixture. Cook until eggs are done, but *not hard*. Turn off the flame. Add grated cheese and cover till melted. Turn out onto plate and garnish with fresh parsley. Beautiful with a sliced ripe pear on the plate. Quick to make but much more interesting than plain eggs.

Liquid Lecithin and Oil

⅔ c. liquid lecithin   ⅓ c. safflower oil

Mix together and put into a storage container. Use to coat the bottom of your pan whenever you cook eggs. When this mixture is used to oil the bottom of your pan for an omelet, it is very healthy and almost guarantees that your omelet will not stick.

Ice Cold Almond Milk

This is delicious for both adults and children who cannot tolerate dairy products. With the new "growth hormones" now given to cows, you might also want to consider this as a healthy alternative to milk for everyday use.

1½ c. raw unsalted almonds   12 c. total of pure water
1 Tbsp. vanilla   large-mouth gallon jar
1 Tbsp. honey or maple syrup   cloth baby diaper
dash of salt   2 lg. strong rubber bands

Put 6 c. water and the almonds into a high-powered blender. Blend on high speed for five minutes, while getting other items ready. Put vanilla and honey in bottom of gallon jar. Make a strainer by placing diaper over top of jar; make a fist and push some of the diaper into the jar, but don't let the edges go into the jar. Put rubber bands around top of jar to hold diaper in place. When blender stops, begin pouring the liquid into the cloth. As it fills up, use a wooden spoon to work the sides of the cloth to get as much of the liquid as possible to pass through the strainer. After putting all the liquid through the cloth, return the pulp to the blender—there is still a lot of nutrients left in the almonds. Add the remaining 6 c. of water and blend again, for a shorter time. When blender becomes slightly warm to the touch, turn it off and put remainder through the cloth. Once you can get no more liquid to pass through, carefully remove the rubber bands. Twist and squeeze the remaining liquid out of the diaper into the jar. Save the pulp for use as bran in muffins, etc. Stir your milk thoroughly. Store in a closed container and refrigerate till very cold. Enjoy over your favorite cold cereal, drink it plain, or cook with it. Our children *love* this!

Cashew Butter

This is a real treat! Use it as you would peanut butter, including in peanut butter cookies.

2 c. raw unsalted cashews   pinch of salt
3 Tbsp. cold-pressed oil, i.e. sesame

Blend nuts at high speed in a high-powered blender until they are as fine as you can get them. Add the oil and salt. Continue blending until very creamy. Stop blender a time or two to scrape the sides. Store in refrigerator and enjoy every bite! Always purchase your nuts from a store that keeps them refrigerated and that sells enough nuts to keep them in fresh supply. When you get them home, always keep them cool. Nuts will become rancid when left in warm temperatures.

SOUPS, SALADS, BISCUITS, AND CORN BREAD
Carrot Dill Soup

1 med. sweet potato   2 Tbsp. unsalted butter
12 carrots, thinly sliced   5 c. broth (i.e., 4 c. water and
1 onion, coarsely chopped   1 can Sheldon's all-natural
1 Tbsp. fresh lemon juice   chicken broth)
1 Irish potato   1/8 c. minced fresh dill

Heat butter in large soup kettle and saute onion over medium heat. Add carrots and soup stock. Bring to a boil, then turn down to simmer. Cut up the rest of the vegetables and add to the pot. Add everything except the dill. Simmer till tender. Next, puree in blender or food processor in batches. Return to pot. Add fresh dill and simmer. If it is too thick, add additional stock, milk, cream, soy milk, etc. Serve hot with a dollop of Alta Dena sour cream, or yogurt and a sprig of fresh dill. Wonderful with honey corn bread and a simple salad.

Cauliflower Soup

1 lg. head cauliflower	1½ c. half-and-half or almond
3 med. potatoes, thinly sliced	milk
1 c. celery, thinly sliced	salt and pepper to taste
1 Tbsp. minced onion	1 Tbsp. chopped parsley
2 Tbsp. butter	4 oz. grated sharp cheddar
2 c. all-natural chicken broth	cheese or soy cheese

Melt butter in sauce pan. Add onion and celery and cook until transparent. Add potatoes and just enough water to cover. Bring to a boil and cook until tender. Do not drain. Cut up cauliflower and cook until tender in a separate pan. Drain. Add cauliflower, broth, cream, and seasoning to potato mixture. Heat, do not boil. Add cheese. Stir until melted. Serve hot.

Millet / Lentil Soup

Part I:	Part II:
1 c. dry millet	1 sm. onion, chopped
1 c. dry lentils	1 grated carrot
5 c. pure water	¼ c. fresh minced parsley
2 tsp. sea salt	2 sm. organic tomatoes
¼ tsp. thyme	1 can Sheldon's all-natural
¼ tsp. oregano	chicken broth

Bring Part I to a boil and simmer for 15 minutes. Add Part II and simmer for 45 minutes, or until lentils are tender. Enjoy with a simple green salad and corn bread.

Quick Corn Chowder

This is so simple and fast you can hardly understand why it would have any flavor. But every time I serve it, people want seconds, especially our children. I think the exceptional flavor can be attributed to the fact that Cascadian Farms produces really tasty organic corn.

2 pkg. Cascadian Farms frozen organic corn	dash of garlic powder (optional)
	½ c. fresh cream (optional)

½ to 1 tsp. Herbamare Seasoning by Bioforce

Put corn in a boiler and barely cover with pure water. Bring to
a boil and simmer for about five minutes. Put in a blender, add
the seasonings, and blend until smooth. Return to boiler and
add cream and simmer until warm again. If you choose not to
use the cream, then when you put it in your bowl it is good with
a dollop of fresh cream on the top. We make this a part of a
quick lunch with hot biscuits and a salad. Of course, fresh corn
is best. It just takes longer. Serves four cups.

Creamy Pea Soup

Once you taste the flavor of organically grown fresh peas, you
probably never will buy any other kind of peas. This recipe is
so easy you can do it blindfolded. But every time I serve it, people
just love it. The fresh mint is very important. It is good served
as a first course.

2 10-oz. pkg Cascadian Farms
frozen organic peas, or home
grown peas

water (barely enough to cover
peas in a boiler)

1 Tbsp. natural vegetable
seasoning

½ c. fresh cream or milk of
your choice (raw cow's,
almond, soy, etc.)

several sprigs of fresh mint (all
supermarkets carry it)

Bring peas to a boil and immediately turn to simmer. Simmer
for five minutes. Turn stove off and let sit for five minutes with
lid on. Blend in blender on high speed. Add your fresh mint and
cream or milk and blend again. Garnish with a tiny spoon of
fresh cream and a small sprig of mint.

Garden Vegetable Stew

1 Tbsp. olive oil
1 onion
2 stalks celery w/leaves
3 carrots
1 turnip
½ sm. head green cabbage
⅓ head cauliflower

1 vegetable bouillon cube (from
health food store)
1 tsp. celery seed
1 tsp. sweet basil
1 tsp. oregano
1 can Sheldon's All-Natural
Chicken Broth

1 sm. bunch broccoli
3 sm. potatoes
½ red pepper
1 zucchini
1 yellow summer squash
1 handful fresh green beans
2 cloves garlic, minced
1 bay leaf

5 c. pure water (depending on
    how thick you like it)
1-2 c. tomato juice
1 c. red chief lentils
1½ c. raw sharp cheddar cheese
    OR 1 c. grated Parmesan cheese
Salt to taste

In large soup pot, saute minced onion in oil, sprinkling salt over the onion to bring out the juices. Add chopped celery and minced garlic and continue cooking. When celery is tender, add liquids and bring to a boil. Begin cutting up vegetables in order listed (hardest vegetables to softest) and add to the pot as soon as they are cut. Add your red chief lentils and all the herbs; stir well and turn down to simmer.

Beautiful Beet Soup

5 lg. organic beets with greens
6 c. soup stock (or water with
    1 heaping Tbsp. all-natural
    bouillon, or 5 c. water and
    1 can Sheldon's all-natural
    chicken broth)
1 onion, finely chopped
1 clove garlic, minced
1 Tbsp. cold-pressed oil
2 carrots, finely chopped
1½ c. chopped red cabbage
2 Tbsp. raw apple cider vinegar

½ lemon, squeezed
1 Tbsp. honey
2 potatoes
½ tsp. caraway seeds
1 can Muir Glen organic crushed
    tomatoes (optional)
Garnish: 1 heaping tsp. Alta
    Dena sour cream, or Brown
    Cow yogurt, or any nondairy
    product, such as tofu sour
    cream, etc.)

In a large soup pot, saute onion in oil; add garlic and simmer a little more. Peel your beets and shred in large shredder; chop the beet greens. Add broth, beets, greens, and carrots; bring to a boil, then simmer while you cut up the rest of your vegetables. Then add all ingredients except honey and simmer until tender (about 30 minutes more). Add honey, stir well, and serve in bowls with your garnish. Excellent with simple green salad and home-made bread. This recipe has delighted more nonbeet-eaters than you can imagine. Our one-year old baby boy loves this blended up in the blender.

Basic Green Salad

Please use all organically grown lettuces. Once you taste the difference, you'll never go back!

1 bunch leafy green lettuce   ½ bunch spinach leaves
1 bunch red leaf lettuce

To this we add different vegetables every meal. OPTIONS: shredded carrots, shredded beets, shredded burdock root, thinly sliced radishes, sliced cucumbers, pumpkin seeds, sunflower seeds, grated cabbage, fresh home-grown sprouts (alfalfa, clover, sunflower, etc.), grated raw cheese, organic boiled eggs, organic garden tomatoes, spring onions. The list is endless—let your imagination be your guide. To this add your favorite homemade dressing. A meal!

Basic Salad Dressing

Put the following ingredients right in the bottom of your salad bowl and mix well with a wire wisk. Then put your greens in, along with whatever else you choose, and toss well with your salad forks.

1 Tbsp. sesame oil (sunflower or   ¼ tsp. mustard
  safflower work well, too)   a little shake of Herbamare by
Just shy of 1 Tbsp. fresh   Bioforce
  squeezed lemon   2 sm. scallions, finely sliced
½ clove crushed garlic

This serves 3 to 4 people. Recipe may be doubled if you need to serve 6.

Sweet and Sour Coleslaw

1 sm. head green cabbage, finely   Dressing:
  shredded   1 Tbsp. raw honey
1 grated carrot   ½ tsp. sea salt
2 Tbsp. chopped celery   1 Tbsp. raw apple cider vinegar
1 Tbsp. chopped green pepper   1 Tbsp. Hain's mayonnaise
1 lg. apple, cored & finely chopped few grains cayenne pepper
1 Tbsp. grated onion

Combine cabbage, carrot, celery, green pepper, apple, and onion in a salad bowl. Beat together the dressing ingredients. Pour over the salad and toss well. Refrigerate at least 20 minutes before serving.

Cucumber Salad

4 cucumbers (organic)
1 tsp. vegetable seasoning
1 Tbsp. raw apple cider vinegar
1 tsp. chopped dill
2 c. plain yogurt

3 Tbsp. olive oil
1 Tbsp. chopped mint
1 clove garlic
Chopped greens to line your
    serving tray

(1) Slice cucumbers and sprinkle with vegetable seasoning. (2) Soak the garlic in vinegar for ten minutes. Strain. (3) Add the dill and vinegar to the yogurt. (4) Add olive oil and mix well. (5) Pour over cucumbers and mix well. (6) Serve on chopped greens and sprinkle with chopped mint.

Zesty Salmon Salad

Everyone knows how to make salmon salad, but for some reason adding a few unusual ingredients makes our children love it.

1 7½-oz. can pink salmon, or
    leftover fresh salmon
1 c. leftover cooked brown rice
3 finely chopped scallions
1 stalk finely chopped celery
¼ c. thinly sliced raw almonds
7 pitted black olives
1 dill pickle, finely chopped
1 Tbsp. dill pickle juice

½ tsp. dried dill
2 or 3 shakes of Worchestershire
    sauce
1-3 tsp. fresh lemon juice (to
    your taste)
2 Tbsp. plain unsweetened yogurt
2 Tbsp. Hain's safflower mayon-
    naise or other good brand
"Sesame Shake" to taste

Mix all ingredients well and refrigerate for at least 30 minutes. Enjoy on a bed of leaf lettuce with whole grain crackers or stuffed in an avocado, garnished with red cherry tomatoes. OPTIONS: You can omit the rice and/or cut in half the amounts of yogurt and mayonnaise. You also can make this with tuna instead of salmon.

Lindsey's Favorite Biscuits

Part I—Dry Ingredients:
1 c. Quinoa flour
1 Tbsp. dry milk powder
1 Tbsp. non-aluminum baking
    powder

Part II—Wet Ingredients:
½ c. milk (raw milk, almond, or
    soy, your choice)
1 egg (nondairy users can sub-
    stitute 1 Tbsp. psyllium husk)

¼ tsp. salt (I substitute Bioforce   2 Tbsp. cold-pressed oil
  Herbamare)

Preheat oven to 425 °F. Mix dry ingredients in stainless steel bowl
and set aside. Mix wet ingredients in a separate bowl. There are
options you may add to wet ingredients before combining the
two bowls. OPTIONS—Choose ONLY ONE: 3 Tbsp. apple
sauce (adjust liquids); ¼ c. grated raw cheddar cheese; 3 Tbsp.
nut butter (Lindsey likes macadamia butter). If you added an
optional ingredient, mix well again. Combine wet and dry ingredients and mix thoroughly. Oil and flour a cookie sheet. Using
a tablespoon, spoon out biscuit mixture onto cookie sheet. Bake
for 12 minutes. Makes 9-12 biscuits. Enjoy while they are hot!
Quinoa is a tasty grain, high in iron, calcium, and fiber.

Honey Corn Bread

1 c. yellow corn meal	1 tsp. baking soda
1 c. whole wheat flour	1 egg
½ tsp. sea salt	1-7/8 c. buttermilk
1 tsp. baking powder	Slightly less than ¼ c. raw honey

Preheat oven to 375 °F. Heavily butter an 8″ × 8″ pan. In a large
bowl, combine the dry ingredients. Stir in the liquid ingredients.
Mix lightly by hand. Corn bread batter must be a little lumpy.
Pour the batter into the prepared pan. Bake for approximately
½ hour, until golden brown. Be sure to test the corn bread by
inserting a toothpick—it should come out clean. VARIATION:
Use ¾ c. yellow corn meal and ¼ c. bran in place of the 1 c.
yellow corn meal.

QUICK LUNCHES

Healthy B.L.T.

The "secret" to this surprise sandwich is the "sesame shake" used
in place of bacon. The first time I served this to my husband,
his eyes got real big and he exclaimed, "Are you feeding me
bacon?" He could not believe it when I told him there was no
bacon in it. We had a good laugh and he's been eating them
ever since.

Whole grain bread slices	Hain's cold-pressed safflower
Organic ripe tomatoes	mayonnaise

Organic lettuce   **Eden brand "Sesame Shake" or homemade (see recipe below)**

Put mayonnaise on both slices of bread, then shake a healthy portion of sesame shake on both slices. Add your lettuce and tomato as usual, assemble, and that's it. The reason I am not suggesting you make your own mayonnaise is because most recipes call for raw egg, and with the wide-spread evidence of salmonella in eggs these days, I am very cautious about making anything with raw eggs now.

Homemade Sesame Shake

sesame seeds   **sea salt**

Simply take some sesame seeds and roast them in a dry frying pan until they are golden and smell nice. Add small amounts of sea salt or "real salt" to your liking. Next, crush them thoroughly using a mortar and pestle. You can use a blender to crush them, but I like doing it by hand. This is a very versatile condiment. We use it nearly everyday on something: vegetables, rice, in soups for flavor, etc. Sesame seeds are the "king" of seeds—full of nutrition!

Children's Cheese, Cucumber, and Lettuce Sandwich

Our daughter loves this sandwich for lunch. It may not suit your children's taste buds yet, but it is worth a try, as it is quite nutritious. Mom likes it too!

Whole grain bread slices   **dash of mustard**
Organic cucumber, thinly sliced   **Raw milk Monterey Jack or**
Organic leaf lettuce   **cheddar cheese slices**
Eden brand sesame shake   **For adults only, a pinch of**
(or homemade)   **horseradish**
Hain's safflower mayonnaise

Arrange bread slices on a cookie sheet and broil one side only until lightly brown. Remove from oven, turn over, and put your cheese slices on half of the number of slices you are broiling. Broil just until cheese is melted. Remove from oven and put a thin coat of mayonnaise, mustard, (and horseradish for adults) on the slices without the cheese. Shake a generous portion of sesame shake also on the slices without the cheese. Next, add your thinly sliced cucumbers and a layer of lettuce leaves, then place bread with the melted cheese on top of each sandwich. Enjoy!

Crunchy Vegetable Sandwich

whole grain bread slices
grated carrot
thinly sliced cucumber
sliced black olives

fresh alfalfa sprouts
Eden's sesame shake
Hain's cold-pressed safflower
  mayonnaise

Put a thin coat of mayonnaise on both slices of your bread and shake with your sesame shake on both slices. (Sesame shake is made from sesame seeds and salt and is very tasty. To make your own at home, see instructions on page 45.) Add all other ingredients in desired order. Enjoy with some Kettle Tias brand five-grain organic chips. My children love this for lunch.

MAIN COURSES AND VEGETABLES

Vegetable Pie

(Fills a 9″ pie crust)

3 lg. organic eggs
1 c. whole milk (or mild soy or
  almond milk)
1 Tbsp. whole wheat flour
¼ tsp. nutmeg
¼ tsp. dry mustard

1 c. grated raw Monterey Jack
  cheese
1 c. grated raw cheddar cheese
¾ c. finely chopped spinach (or
  vegetables of choice)

Preheat oven to 350°F. Combine eggs, milk, flour, nutmeg, and mustard in blender. Fill unbaked whole wheat pie shell with the grated cheese. Top with spinach. OPTIONS: you may substitute or add to the spinach a combination of yellow squash, green and yellow onions, and red pepper in winter is fun; broccoli and cauliflower are good, or whatever you have left over. Pour blended ingredients over the top and bake for about 1 hour, or until set and lightly brown on top. If any of your vegetables are sticking up above the liquid, it is important to cover your pie pan with another pie pan while cooking so that they do not burn or get hard and dry.

Organic Meat Pie

1 lb. organic ground beef, turkey, or lamb	1 tsp. oregano
1 sm. onion	1 tsp. sweet basil
1 bunch broccoli, steamed	¼ tsp. dry mustard
1 organic ripe tomato, finely chopped and seeded	1 Tbsp. tamari sauce or Braggs liquid aminos
3 lg. eggs	1 squirt of Worcestershire sauce
1 c. raw milk (or soy, almond, etc.)	1½ c. grated raw cheddar cheese
1 Tbsp. whole wheat flour	(or nondairy cheese)

Preheat oven to 350°F. Fill the bottom of your unbaked pie crust with the cheese. Brown your meat with the onion in a fry pan and drain the grease very well. Place half of the meat in pie shell on top of the cheese. Then place half the broccoli and half the tomato on top of the meat. Next, add layers of the remaining meat, broccoli, and tomato. Blend all remaining ingredients in a blender and pour mixture over meat and vegetables. Cover with second half of rolled dough and flute the edges OR cover with another pie pan to prevent drying out. Bake for about 1 hour or until set and lightly brown on top. Let cool slightly before serving—it will cut better. Very nice for special occasions or company who thinks they don't like "health food."

Medley of Stir-Fry Vegetables

1 heaping Tbsp. sesame oil	1 c. celery, cut diagonally
1 bunch broccoli	½ lg. red pepper, cut in strips
½ head cauliflower	3 carrots, cut diagonally
1 med. onion	1 yellow squash, sliced
3 cloves garlic, minced	1 can water chestnuts, sliced
1 c. fresh snow peas	any other vegetables you wish

Put sesame oil into your wok and let it get hot. Add hardest vegetables first, such as carrots, and add others as you go along. A nice addition right at the end is a large handful of mung bean sprouts. Season with mineral salt, tamari sauce, and herbs of your choice. The organic vegetables have such a nice flavor that you don't have to use much seasoning. Serve over brown rice and with a simple green salad. Delicious!

Basic Brown Rice

2 c. brown rice (long grain is   4 c. pure water
nice in summer, short grain in   1 tsp. salt
winter)

Put in large stainless steel pan and bring to a boil. Simmer for
about one hour. It should soak up all the water, but still be chewy,
not mushy. If your burner is turned up too high, you will run
out of water and have to add more. Brown rice will nourish your
family and give them strength, while white rice has much of the
nutrients removed.

Tangy Stir-Fry Sauce

½ c. orange juice   2-3 cloves garlic, minced
¼ c. Braggs aminos or tamari   1-2 Tbsp. raw honey
sauce   2 tsp. toasted sesame oil
1 Tbsp. grated fresh ginger   2 Tbsp. cornstarch

Combine the first six ingredients. Put the cornstarch in a bowl
and whisk the liquid mixture into it. Set it aside. Once the
vegetables in your wok are about two-thirds cooked, then whisk
the liquid mixture again and add it to the wok. Stir from the
bottom constantly so all the vegetables get coated, and so it won't
stick to the bottom. Scrumptious!

Pecan and Tofu Herb Loaf

½ onion, finely chopped   4 Tbsp. nutritional yeast
1 Tbsp. cold-pressed olive oil   1½ tsp. salt
8 med. mushrooms, finely   ¼ tsp. ground black pepper
chopped   ½ tsp. basil
3-4 garlic cloves, finely chopped   ¼ tsp. oregano
½ c. pecans, raw   ¼ tsp. savory
½ c. almonds, raw   ¼ tsp. garlic powder
¼ c. chia seeds (or ½ c. sesame   20 oz. firm organic Tofu (this is
seeds)   MORE than one cake of Tofu)
2 Tbsp. soy flour   5 Tbsp. raw tahini (sesame
2 Tbsp. arrowroot powder (a   butter)
thickener)

Preheat oven to 350°F. Saute the onion in oil over medium heat
for 3 minutes. Add the mushrooms and cover; cook for 5 min.

Add the garlic and cook another 2 minutes.

Place pecans and almonds in a food processor or blender. Using short strokes at medium speed, chop the nuts until they have the texture of very course corn meal.

Combine the nuts, chia seeds, soy flour, arrowroot, yeast, salt, pepper, basil, oregano, savory, and garlic powder in a large mixing bowl and mix well.

Drain Tofu well. Break into small pieces and combine thoroughly with the onion mushroom mixture and tahini. Add to dry ingredients and combine well with your hands. Press firmly into covered casserole dish (oiled) and bake for 1 hour. Remove from oven and let sit for 15 minutes. Turn out onto a serving dish and cover with mushroom sauce and garnish with sprigs of fresh parsley. This is good for a party, as it is very elegant, though a bit time consuming.

Marvelous Mushroom Sauce

This is excellent over the Pecan and Tofu Herb Loaf, brown rice, or vegetables.

1 Tbsp. olive oil	1 Tbsp. soy sauce
½ onion, finely chopped	1 tsp. Worcestershire sauce
¼ tsp. salt	2 tsp. arrowroot
1 clove garlic, finely chopped	¼ tsp. paprika
6 med. mushrooms, sliced	pepper to taste
1 c. almond milk, soy, etc.	3 Tbsp. fresh parsley

OPTION: For special occasions you can add 2 Tbsp. red wine. The alcohol will cook out of the sauce in the cooking.

Mix arrowroot with a little cold water and set aside. Heat the oil in a saucepan and add the onion. Sprinkle salt over the onion, cover, and cook over medium heat until the onion is golden. The salt will release the juices from the onion and it will stew in its own juice. Add the garlic and mushroom. Cook covered for 3 minutes. Add all other ingredients and cook covered for 20 minutes longer. If it becomes too thick, you can add a little water to thin it out. Enjoy!

Bean Burritos Supreme

4½ c. water	1½ c. dry beans, soaked over-

night (black beans or pinto
beans)

Cook above for one to two hours, until tender. OPTION:
Attention Busy Ladies! Try Taste Adventure brand precooked
instant black bean flakes instead of dry beans. Follow directions.

Now put your cooked beans in a food processor or blender
and add:

½ minced onion, sauteed   1 Tbsp. tamari sauce or Bragg's
½ tsp. chili powder   aminos
¼ tsp. cayenne pepper

Blend well until it makes a paste.

Now arrange the following on a table:

½ minced onion   6 all-natural Chapatis (whole
2 organic tomatoes, chopped   wheat tortillas)
  into small pieces in small bowl 3 cloves minced garlic in 3 Tbsp.
1 c. grated raw cheddar cheese in olive oil in small bowl
  small bowl   1 dish of all-natural salsa

Assemble each burrito in the following order: (1) Using a pastry
brush, put a light coat of the olive oil/garlic mixture on each
tortilla. (2) Spread 1 Tbsp. salsa in middle of tortilla and spread
around, using circular motion. (3) Sprinkle minced onions on
each tortilla. (4) Sprinkle tomatoes on each tortilla. (5) Sprinkle
cheese on each tortilla. (6) Put heaping Tbsp. of bean mixture
on each tortilla, kind of a strip down the center. Fold the two
sides over and flip over and place on cookie sheet.

Heat in oven at 350°F for 10 to 15 minutes, only until warm
and the cheese melts. Do not let tortilla get hard. Place on plate
and garnish with avocado, sour cream, and black olives. Serve
with shredded lettuce on ⅓ of the plate and brown rice rice on
⅓ of the plate. Festive!

Lemon Herb Chicken

1 lemon, squeezed   garlic powder
1 skinless, boneless chicken breast seasoned salt, with herbs
¼ stick of butter   salt to taste

Squeeze lemon and put in stainless steel bowl. Immerse chicken
in lemon juice for 15 minutes. Heat electric frying pan to 400°F

and melt butter in pan. Put chicken breast in for 5 minutes. Turn over and cook another 5 minutes. Turn temperature down to 300°F. Pour excess lemon juice over breast, season with the spices. Cover and cook for an additional 10 minutes. SERVING SUGGESTIONS: cut up finely in stir-fry vegetables or served on its own with a bed of brown, wild rice, vegetables, and a salad.

Austrian Potato Salad

2 c. cubed, cooked potatoes	2 oz. raw apple cider vinegar
2 c. cubed, unpeeled raw apples	1 Tbsp. vegetable broth powder
2 oz. cold-pressed, unheated	3 sliced, hard-boiled eggs for
vegetable oil (sesame is good)	garnish

(1) Mix potatoes and apples together. (2) Create a dressing from the oil, vinegar, and vegetable broth powder, using a wire wisk. (3) Garnish with slices of hard-boiled eggs. This recipe is so simple, yet every time I serve it, I get raving reviews!

Butternut Squash with Pecans

3 med. butternut squash	2 Tbsp. raw honey
1½ c. raw pecans	dash of cinnamon

Cut each squash in half and cook in large covered casserole dish in oven, with about an inch of water in the bottom of the dish. Cook at 400°F for about 30-45 minutes, until soft. At the same time, take a cookie sheet and butter the bottom. Place your raw pecans on the cookie sheet and salt a little. Put in oven with the squash, but only for about 10 minutes until golden and they smell good. Once squash is done, scoop it out of its shells and into a nice serving dish. Sprinkle the roasted pecans all over the top. Slightly warm your honey and dribble over entire creation. Sprinkle with cinnamon and serve. Recently I served this with the Austrian Potato Salad and a green salad, and it was a big hit.

DESSERTS

Organic Peach or Blueberry Pie

Make one 9″ pie or tart

4 c. organic peaches or	¼ c. unbleached flour
blueberries	½ tsp. cinnamon

2 Tbsp. fresh lemon juice   ½ tsp. allspice
⅓ c. raw unprocessed honey   1 Tbsp. arrowroot

Preheat oven to 400°F. In a small bowl, combine honey, flour,
spices, and arrowroot. Mix with fork until well blended. In a
large bowl, toss together fruit and lemon juice. Gently fold honey
mixture into fruit mixture. Set aside while preparing your dough,
if it is not already made. (The Almond Pecan Nut Crust is
wonderful for this—see next recipe.) Pour into your pie shell.
Cover with your top pie shell and flute the edges, or bake it
without a crust on top (a tart). If you do not use a top crust,
cover the pie with another pie tin while baking to prevent the
fruit from drying out. Bake for 50-55 minutes until the crust
is golden brown. Let settle for 2 to 3 hours before serving in
order to set firm. We love it with honey vanilla ice cream.

Almond Pecan Nut Crust

Makes one 9″ unbaked crust

¾ c. finely minced almonds and   4 Tbsp. cold butter, cut into
  pecans (just this side of   small pieces
  "ground")   1 c. organic unbleached flour
dash of salt   3-5 Tbsp. cold water

Put nuts, butter, flour, and salt together in a bowl. Use a pastry
cutter to work the mixture until it is uniform and resembles a
coarse corn meal. Gradually drizzle in the cold water and begin
using a fork. Mix by pushing the dough into itself in the center
of the bowl. When the dough adheres to itself, you've added
enough water. Roll out the dough and fit it into your oiled pie
pan. Cover with waxed paper and chill until time to fill. Tasty
when used for a carrot pie or peach or blueberry tart.

Italian Cream Cake

This recipe is adapted from my mother's cook book, *The Mousse
and Me*. It is a healthier version, but still reminds me of all the
special birthday parties our mom planned when we were children.
The flavor is exactly the same!

5 organic eggs, separated (room 2 tsp. vanilla
  temperature)   2 c. organic unbleached flour

2 c. Sucanat®, finely sifted
1 stick butter
¼ c. cold-pressed oil
1½ c. buttermilk

1 tsp. baking soda
½ c. unsweetened shredded
  coconut
1 c. chopped pecans

Preheat oven to 350°F. Beat 5 egg whites until soft peaks form. Gradually add ¼ c. Sucanat® (which you have sifted fine in your flour sifter), beating until stiff. Cream together the remaining 1¾ c. Sucanat®, oil, butter, and egg yolks. Combine the buttermilk and 1 tsp. of the vanilla. In another bowl, combine the flour and baking soda. Alternately add the buttermilk mixture and flour mixture to the creamed mixture. Gently fold egg whites into batter, adding remaining vanilla. Fold in the coconut and pecans. Grease and flour three 9″ round cake pans. Fill the pans and bake for 25 minutes. Frost with Cream Cheese Honey Frosting (see next recipe).

Simple Cream Cheese Frosting

16 oz. cream cheese (Alta Dena
  is a good brand)
¼ c. butter

1 tsp. natural vanilla extract
½ c. raw honey (a light-colored
  honey works best for this)

Whip ingredients with beaters or in a food processor until smooth. Spread on cake of your choice just before serving. Children don't even miss the taste of the unhealthy sugar frostings because this is very satisfying.

Carob Cake

2 c. unbleached white flour
1 c. carob powder
2 Tbsp. instant coffee or natural
  coffee flavor
1 tsp. baking soda
1 tsp. baking powder

¾ c. melted butter
1½ tsp. pure vanilla extract
1½ c. ice water
1 c. chopped nuts (optional)
3 eggs
1¾ c. honey

Preheat oven to 350°F. Oil a 9″ × 13″ baking pan and set aside. Sift together the dry ingredients. Beat the eggs in a separate bowl. Blend in the honey, melted butter, and vanilla and beat thoroughly. Add the wet ingredients alternately with the ice water to the dry ingredients. Beat until smooth. The batter will be quite thin. Fold in the nuts, if desired. Pour the batter into the pan and bake 30 to 40 minutes, until a knife inserted in the middle comes out clean. Frost with a cream cheese or whipped cream frosting.

Pumpkin Muffins

These muffins are a special treat at Thanksgiving. If you want to have something around other than just pumpkin pie, give them a try. They are very moist and they make a huge batch. Children and grandchildren love them!

3⅓ c. whole wheat pastry flour	⅔ c. water
2 c. pumpkin puree	2 tsp. baking soda
2-3 finely grated carrots	1 tsp. cinnamon
3 c. pure maple syrup	1 tsp. nutmeg
4 eggs	½ tsp. ginger
1 c. cold-pressed oil	½ tsp. allspice
1 c. chopped nuts	2 tsp. salt
½ c. raisins	

Preheat oven to 350°F. Sift all dry ingredients together. Make a "well" in the middle and add all the wet ingredients. Mix well. Add nuts, raisins, and carrots. Put into greased muffin cups. Bake for about 15 minutes. Delicious with a little real butter on them.

Christmas Peanut Butter Balls

This recipe comes from my dear sister Kathy. Growing up, she made dozens of these every Christmas for us all to enjoy. They were her favorites.

½ c. peanut butter (healthy brand with NO added sugar)	2 Tbsp. sesame seeds or chopped peanuts
½ c. wheat germ	carob chips, sweetened with corn and barley malt
½ c. nonfat dry milk	
½ c. raw unprocessed honey	

Mix and chill. Then roll into balls and freeze. Dip balls into melted carob chips (sweetened with corn and barley malt), or if you absolutely do not like carob, then use semisweet chocolate chips. Store in refrigerator. Makes 24 balls. This is a healthy Christmas treat for children and adults alike. Also, we love to make them with almond butter or cashew butter, instead of peanut butter for a change.

Natural Peanut Butter Cookies

This dough is rather stiff, so it requires a good strong mixer.

Mix:
1 c. peanut butter
½ c. butter or ¼ c. oil
1 c. Sucanat® (sifted in your
  flour sifter); use less if you do
  not like them too sweet
½ c. honey
2 eggs

Add:
2½ c. whole wheat pastry flour
1 tsp. baking powder
1 tsp. baking soda
½ tsp. salt

Roll into balls and press with a floured fork, as you would any
peanut butter cookie. You may have to refrigerate for 30 minutes
if dough is too soft. Bake for 8-10 minutes. Do not overbake.
They should be chewy. OPTION: Add one cup unsweetened
carob chips at the end. This is our family's favorite cookie. Also,
we often make them with almond butter or macadamia butter
instead of peanut butter.

Best Oatmeal Cookies

Cream the following ingredients:

1 c. butter (or ½ c. oil)
1 c. raw unprocessed honey

1 tsp. vanilla
1 egg

Sift the following ingredients:

1½ c. organic whole wheat
  pastry flour

1 tsp. cinnamon
2 tsp. baking powder

Mix wet and dry ingredients (above) thoroughly, then add:

2½ c. oats
½ c. wheat germ (¾ c. if your
  honey is the really thin kind)

1 c. total of the following (single
  or combined): dates,
  unsweetened carob chips,
  raisins, or chopped nuts

Drop onto oiled cookie sheet and bake at 350°F for 8-10 minutes.
Enjoy!